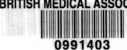

MCQ Companion to the Eye

Basic Sciences in Practice

To Janet, Lucy and Matthew

Commissioning Editor: Michael Parkinson
Project Development Manager: Lynn Watt
Project Controller: Nancy Arnott
Designer: Erik Bigland

MCQ Companion to the Eye

Basic Sciences in Practice

Peter H. Galloway

Specialist Registrar in Ophthalmology
South West Rotation
UK

John V. Forrester

Professor of Ophthalmology
and Head of Department of Ophthalmology
University of Aberdeen

Andrew D. Dick

Professor of Ophthalmology
and Head of Division of Ophthalmology
University of Bristol

William R. Lee

Formerly Professor of Ocular Pathology
University of Glasgow

 W.B. SAUNDERS

EDINBURGH • LONDON • NEW YORK • PHILADELPHIA • ST LOUIS
SYDNEY • TORONTO 2001

WB SAUNDERS
An imprint of Harcourt Publishers Limited

© Harcourt Publishers Limited 2001

 is a registered trademark of Harcourt Publishers Limited

First published 2001

ISBN 0 702 025666

British Library Cataloguing in Publication Data
A catalogue record for this book is available from the British Library

Library of Congress Cataloging in Publication Data
A catalog record for this book is available from the Library of Congress

Note
Medical knowledge is constantly changing. As new information becomes available,
changes in treatment, procedures, equipment and the use of drugs become
necessary. The editors/authors/contributors and the publishers have, as far as it is
possible, taken care to ensure that the information given in this text is accurate
and up to date. However, readers are strongly advised to confirm that the
information, especially with regard to drug usage, complies with
the latest legislation and standards of practice.

Printed in China

Preface

This first edition of a multiple choice book to accompany *The Eye: Basic Sciences in Practice* provides sets of questions aimed at basic science examinations in ophthalmology. The questions are organized into 4 sections, consisting of 60 stem questions each. Overall the sections have been designed to provide an appropriate balance for all key subjects including anatomy, embryology, microbiology, pathology, biochemistry, immunology, physiology, genetics, pharmacology and statistics.

For those not familiar with the details of the technique of answering MCQs, the style of each question is in a standard true false format. Five independent statements follow each stem question, and each statement requires a true or false answer. Incorrect answers forfeit a mark but those left blank carry no penalty.

Candidates are encouraged to sit each paper as a whole, and time themselves accordingly to exam specifications. Brief explanations are provided within this book; however, for a deeper understanding of any topic, the companion textbook and others referenced will provide a more in-depth discussion. Readers are encouraged to look up not just incorrect answers but also correct responses where the suspicion of guesswork is involved.

Strategy and technique in examinations with a negative marking system is important, and is dependent in particular on the reader's overall level of confidence in responding true or false over opting out and responding `don't know'. With a negative marking system, guessing is a less productive option if the degree of certainty on a question is close to 50:50. If this strategy is repeated there is a risk of being unlucky and obtaining an overall poor score by chance. Yet it is essential to make educated or informed guesses. In reality it is difficult to be absolutely confident about many responses, particularly in an exam setting. Many questions involve making some connection between threads of knowledge covering several subject areas; if you can develop a rational explanation for an answer that seems logical *then mark a true or false response* as otherwise there may be a risk of not answering enough questions to pass the examination.

For those wishing to receive an automated breakdown of performance by subject, with an overall percent score for their attempt, readers are directed to www.vision-capture.com to download instructions and a response sheet. This will generate an anonymous and confidential reply indicating performance by category as illustrated in Figure 1 below.

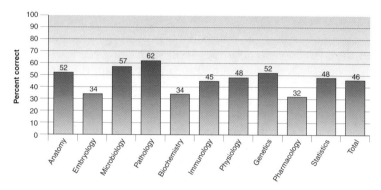

Fig. 1   Sample breakdown of results by subject.

Peter H. Galloway
West of England Eye Unit
Exeter, UK

Contents

Questions

Paper 1	1
Paper 2	17
Paper 3	33
Paper 4	49

Answers

Paper 1	65
Paper 2	85
Paper 3	105
Paper 4	123

Bibliography	143
Index	145

Paper 1 – Questions

QUESTIONS

1. **The oculomotor nerve:**

   a   is connected to the fourth and sixth cranial nerves by the medial longitudinal fasciculus
   b   passes medial to the posterior communicating artery
   c   if cut results in complete ptosis
   d   contains parasympathetic fibres lying central in the nerve
   e   lies in apposition to the internal carotid artery in the cavernous sinus

2. **The superior orbital fissure:**

   a   lies between the lesser and greater wings of the sphenoid
   b   is widest laterally
   c   transmits the upper division of the oculomotor nerve through the common tendinous ring
   d   transmits the nasociliary nerve below the common tendinous ring
   e   lies between the roof and the medial wall of the orbit

3. **The corneal epithelium:**

   a   has superficial cells which contain no nucleus
   b   is about 200 µm thick
   c   has a glycocalyx
   d   is linked to Bowman's layer by a basement membrane
   e   contains melanin centrally

4. ***Staphylococcus aureus*:**

   a   produces blue colonies on chocolate agar
   b   is usually penicillin resistant
   c   produces an enterotoxin
   d   is a well recognized cause of endocarditis
   e   is a commensal of the nasal mucosa in over 30% of the population

5. Roundworm infestation:

a is classified into tissue and intestinal forms
b associated with deer fly is called *Trichinella spiralis*
c associated with black fly is diagnosed by skin biopsy
d transmitted from pigs is caused by *Enterobius vermicularis*
e transmitted from dogs is called *Toxocara canis*

6. The cornea contains:

a collagen fibres embedded in glycosaminoglycans
b abundant glycosaminoglycans, predominantly hyaluronic acid
c an abundance of type II collagen in Bowman's layer
d interdigitating 'wing' cells within the epithelial layer
e a subepithelial nerve plexus

7. The cavernous sinus:

a contains the internal carotid artery, which travels with the sixth cranial nerve
b is traversed by the maxillary nerve within the inferolateral wall
c receives blood directly from the inferior petrosal sinus
d contains cranial nerves III and V in the lateral wall
e lies anterior to the optic chiasm

8. The right fourth nerve nucleus:

a lies in the rostral pons
b gives rise to fibres that innervate the right superior oblique
c gives rise to the trochlear nerve which passes above the third nerve
d contains over 20 000 fibres
e crosses the roof of the brainstem

9. Corneal endothelial cells:

a form a specialized squamous layer
b rest on Desçemet's membrane
c are interdigitating
d amount to about 800 cells per square millimetre at birth
e form a hexagonal array

10. **The following are paired venous sinuses:**

    a transverse
    b straight
    c occipital
    d petrosal
    e basilar

11. **The sclera:**

    a has a higher glycosaminoglycan content than the cornea
    b is avascular
    c is thinnest at the posterior pole
    d consists mainly of collagen type II
    e has a similar water content to the cornea

12. **In ciliary body development:**

    a growth starts around the same time as the lens
    b *Hox* gene expression is restricted to the inner
      pigmented layer of the developing neuroectoderm
    c aqueous is produced from 20 weeks' gestation onwards
    d ciliary muscle develops from mesenchyme
    e radial ciliary muscle fibres develop before circular fibres

13. **The limbus:**

    a is 3.0–4.0 mm in width
    b has a V-shaped corneal termination
    c receives the termination of Bowman's layer and
      Descemet's membrane
    d has an anterior margin formed by the junction between
      corneal and conjunctival epithelium
    e has a posterior margin formed by an artificial line
      which passes through the scleral spur

14. ***Clostridium botulinum*:**

    a is a spore-forming anaerobe
    b produces a toxin which interferes with release of
      acetylcholine from the motor nerve terminal
    c directly binds to motor endplates
    d infection is most commonly due to types F and G
    e causes fever

15. The optic nerve:

    a intracranially is 4 cm long
    b contains first order neurones
    c is superior to the anterior part of the cavernous sinus
    d contains approximately 1.2 million axons
    e receives its blood supply via the pial vessel network

16. The lateral geniculate bodies:

    a lie superior to the thalamus
    b contain six layers, the first layer containing fibres derived from the ipsilateral eye
    c contain mostly macula-derived fibres
    d have input from areas 17, 18, and 19 of striate cortex
    e project to areas 17, 18, and 19 of striate cortex

17. Bruch's membrane:

    a is a cellular connective tissue layer
    b is a single layer of basement membrane
    c is about 300 nm thick
    d contains a central elastic zone
    e consists of inner and outer collagenous zones

18. In the 6-week-old embryo:

    a the optic chiasm is fully formed
    b myelination of the optic nerve begins
    c retinal differentiation starts
    d primary lens fibres are first manufactured
    e the fetal fissure forms

19. The following are derived from the 1st pharyngeal arch:

    a malleus bone
    b greater horn of hyoid bone
    c thyroid cartilage
    d arytenoid cartilage
    e stylopharyngeus

20. Crystallins in lens cells:

a   are insoluble proteins
b   are coded for by a single chromosome
c   are related to heat shock proteins
d   if deficient cause cataracts in mice
e   account for the expansion and lengthening of secondary lens fibres

21. Concerning the iris:

a   it is unique in that its muscles arise directly from neuroectoderm
b   the dilator muscle develops as an extension from the posterior epithelium
c   it contains melanocytes which complete their migration 2 weeks postpartum
d   during development the anterior epithelial layer loses pigment
e   it may not form if the short arm of chromosome 17 is deleted

22. Components of the vitreous include:

a   ascorbate
b   lipids
c   collagen type II
d   70% water
e   non-sulphated glycosaminoglycans

23. The orbital margin:

a   is formed by four bones
b   is thickest superiorly
c   has a sharp distinct lower medial border
d   is formed by the maxilla inferolaterally
e   is concave laterally

24. The following structures form part of the midbrain:

a   fifth cranial nerve nucleus
b   red nucleus
c   nucleus ambiguus
d   Edinger–Westphal nucleus
e   vertical gaze centre

25. In diabetic microangiopathy:

a usually the basement membrane of the retinal capillaries is thickened
b capillary pericyte loss is typical
c microaneurysms contain PAS-positive material
d intraretinal microvascular anomalies leak proteins
e hard exudates form at the level of the inner plexiform layer

26. The first division of the trigeminal nerve:

a is the largest division
b runs in the lateral wall of the cavernous sinus below the trochlear nerve
c divides into two branches
d gives rise to the lacrimal nerve, which enters the orbit below the annulus of Zinn
e supplies the skin of the lower part of the nose

27. The meibomian glands:

a are large sebaceous glands
b form a double row on the lower eyelid
c are more common in the lower eye-lid than in the upper
d secrete fatty acids and cholesterol
e contain ducts lined by a single layer of cuboidal cells

28. Branches of the internal carotid artery include:

a the posterior communicating artery
b the anterior cerebral artery
c the middle cerebral artery
d the ophthalmic artery
e the submaxillary artery

29. Metastases can occur in the following tissue layers:

a peritoneum
b subarachnoid space
c pericardium
d conjunctival epithelium
e lens epithelium

30. **Dystrophic calcification can occur within:**

    a the media of blood vessels
    b the corneal stroma
    c the normal epididymis
    d tuberculous lymph nodes
    e necrotic tumour tissue

31. **In various forms of embolic disease the pulmonary arterioles may contain:**

    a fat cells
    b amniotic squames
    c splenic cells
    d *Pneumocystis carinii*
    e adenocarcinoma

32. **The following cells participate in allograft rejection:**

    a eosinophil polymorphonuclear leucocytes
    b CD4 T lymphocytes
    c CD8 T lymphocytes
    d platelets
    e mast cells

33. **In a fracture in a bone it is possible to identify:**

    a rhabdomyoblasts
    b lamellar bone
    c woven bone
    d chondrocytes
    e Purkinje cells

34. **In pathological states the following may be deposited in the extracellular matrix:**

    a ferric salts
    b lipofuscin
    c calcium salts
    d glycosaminoglycans
    e RNA

35. The following tumours have the capacity to metastasize to distant sites:

a squamous cell carcinoma
b pituitary adenoma
c choroidal melanoma
d retinoblastoma
e capillary haemangioma

36. In ischaemia the following tissue components are identified:

a amyloid deposits
b plasma exudates
c keratin
d budding endothelial cells
e macrophages containing iron

37. Irradiation therapy causes:

a loss of pilosebaceous follicles
b chromosomal fragmentation
c increased mitotic activity
d increased depostion of brown fat
e endarteritis

38. Regarding features of pharyngeal arch development:

a they subserve cranial nerves III, VII, IX and X
b arch 1 cleft ectoderm forms the outer ear
c arch 2 forms Meckel's cartilage (malleus bone)
d arch 2 forms part of the digastric muscle
e arch 6 forms the extrinsic muscles of the larynx

39. α-Adrenergic blocking agents:

a have profound effects on blood pressure
b increase sympathetic tone in peripheral blood vessels
c affect β receptors in the heart
d may induce reflex tachycardia
e aggravate asthma

40. The following structures lie posterior to the grey line of the eyelid:

a crypts of Henle
b meibomian glands
c glands of Wolfring
d glands of Moll
e lash follicles

41. The arterial supply to the retina:

a is derived from two sources
b forms arteriovenous anastamoses
c drains via the central vein of the retina
d follows a similar pattern to lymphatic vessels
e forms a capillary-free zone about 200 μm in diameter

42. The roof of the fourth ventricle is formed by:

a superior cerebellar peduncles
b superior medullary velum
c inferior medullary velum
d pia mater
e inferior cerebellar peduncles

43. With regard to ocular neovascularization:

a vascular endothelial growth factor (VEGF) is expressed on retinal capillary endothelial cells
b corticosteroid therapy may induce regression of new vessels
c neovascularization is pathognomonic of diabetic retinopathy
d neovascularization may occur as a result of ocular inflammation
e neovascularization in diabetics is associated with a high concentration of vascular endothelial growth factor within the vitreous

44. The hyaloid artery:

a develops in concert with the hyaloid vein
b regresses in the second trimester
c is patent and connected to the optic disk at month 7
d may persist as a remnant at the optic disk, named as 'Morning Glory syndrome'
e develops branches that form the central retinal artery

45. Benign tumours that form within epithelial tissue feature:

a basophilic cells in basal cell papilloma
b keratin cysts in basal cell papilloma
c rapid growth in keratoacanthoma
d cytoplasmic inclusions in molluscum contagiosum
e a palpable raised border in a junctional naevus

46. Regarding laboratory tests in human immunodeficiency virus (HIV) infection:

a HIV may be isolated by co-culture with lymphocytes in the presence of interleukin-2
b Western blots identify retroviral ribonucleic acid (RNA)
c p24 antigenaemia precedes the antibody response by about 3 weeks
d the polymerase chain reaction (PCR) detects nucleic acids
e antibody to HIV-1 may be detected by enzyme-linked immunosorbent assay (ELISA)

47. Examples of viruses that contain ribonucleic acid (RNA) include:

a human immunodeficiency virus
b *Arenavirus*
c *Rhinovirus*
d togavirus
e papovavirus

48. **Botulinum toxin type A:**

   a acts postsynaptically at the motor endplate
   b induces sprouting of nerve terminals as a consequence of paralysis
   c prevents release of cholinergic vesicles
   d is a competitive inhibitor of acetylcholine release from nerve terminals
   e is one of eight serotypes

49. **Chronic inflammation:**

   a usually results from prolonged acute inflammatory change
   b if non-granulomatous is typified by epithelioid cells and polymorphs
   c if granulomatous is typified by plasma cells and lymphocytes
   d produces a diffuse granulomatous response in sarcoid
   e features Touton giant cells associated with lipid disorders such as juvenile xanthogranuloma

50. *Acanthamoeba*:

   a requires selective culture with streptococcus-enriched agar
   b is stained with calcafluor white
   c is a free-living organism
   d is known to cause a granulomatous encephalitis
   e produces trophozoites and cysts which are identifiable on biopsy

51. *Chlamydia trachomatis*:

   a is Gram-negative
   b can make ATP
   c does not have a peptidoglycan cell wall and is therefore susceptible to beta-lactam antibiotics
   d contains eosinophilic cytoplasmic inclusion bodies
   e is classified by indirect immunofluorescence

52. Dense regular connective tissue contains:

a fibroblasts
b abundant extracellular fibres
c abundant cells
d amorphous ground substance
e abundant collagen fibres

53. The transport of molecules across the lens surface:

a primarily utilizes the Na^+/K^+ ATPase pump within the lens epithelium
b utilizes specific glucose transporters
c utilizes specific ascorbate transporters
d including chloride and water involves an active transport mechanism
e requires the Na^+/K^+ ATPase pump to import Na^+ ions from the aqueous

54. Levator palpebrae superioris:

a forms the medial palpebral ligament from its medial horn
b originates from the greater wing of the sphenoid bone
c lies below the superior rectus
d is about 4 cm long
e usually is capable of raising the upper lid by 5 mm at the most

55. In response to infection or inflammation, the acquired immune system includes:

a the mucosa-associated immune system
b lymphocyte-secreted cytokines
c phagocytic and cytotoxic cells, for example eosinophils
d macrophage tumour necrosis factor
e dendritic cells

56. The central retinal artery:

   a is an end artery
   b is not a true 'artery'
   c usually divides into two branches at the optic disk
   d accompanies a vein
   e is the second branch of the ophthalmic artery

57. Optic nerve glioma:

   a exists in juvenile and adult forms
   b usually displaces the globe upwards
   c is bilateral in 30% of cases
   d contains psammoma bodies
   e contains Flexner–Wintersteiner rosettes

58. Acute inflammatory processes:

   a usually begin within minutes of an insult
   b are predominantly mediated by neutrophils after 24 hours
   c when affecting the eye lead to clinical lymphadenopathy
   d start with leucocyte adhesion then margination
   e are usually protective responses, except in the eye

59. The tear film:

   a is about 100 μm thick
   b contains mucin secreted by conjunctival goblet cells
   c acts to smooth out reticulations of the epithelial surface
   d contains a thick lipid layer
   e contains IgM and IgG

60. A polymorphonuclear leucocytic infiltrate is a feature of infection by:

   a herpes simplex
   b herpes zoster
   c *Acanthamoeba*
   d *Streptococcus pyogenes*
   e mucormycosis

Paper 2 – Questions

QUESTIONS

1. **Glutamate:**

   a is the major neurotransmitter released from
      photoreceptors
   b inhibits NMDA receptors
   c is a complex amino acid
   d is inhibitory to horizontal cells
   e binds to receptors which open ion channels

2. **The following diseases are inherited in an X-linked fashion:**

   a oculocutaneous albinism
   b retinitis pigmentosa type 3
   c choroideraemia
   d Norrie's disease
   e Fabry's disease

3. **G proteins:**

   a are second messengers
   b may decrease calcium stores
   c bind to rhodopsin
   d interact with adenylate cyclase
   e are thought to play a role in intraocular pressure
      control

4. **The following are features of mitochondrial diseases:**

   a sons of probands usually transmit the disease
   b Leber's hereditary optic neuropathy is the
      prototype
   c females are predominantly affected
   d 'ragged red fibres' may be found on muscle biopsy
   e tissues and organs least reliant on mitochondria, such
      as the kidney and endocrine organs, are paradoxically
      affected worst by the disease process

5. **The innervation of the lacrimal apparatus:**

   a is derived from the pterygopalatine ganglion, which provides sympathetic and parasympathetic fibres
   b is derived from the pons
   c would be interrupted by a lesion affecting the greater petrosal nerve
   d is derived from the retro-orbital plexus
   e is predominantly sympathetic in origin

6. **The structure of the tear film:**

   a includes an inner lipid layer
   b is formed in part by an aqueous layer secreted mainly by the lacrimal glands of Krause and Wolfring
   c contains a mucin layer, which is secreted by the goblet cells, with a minor contribution from the crypts of Henle and the glands of Manz
   d is disrupted usually about 12 to 15 times a minute
   e contains secretory IgA, which is highest in concentration in nonstimulated tears

7. **Toxic effects of aminoglycoside antibiotics include:**

   a ototoxicity when given systemically
   b retinal necrosis
   c an extinguished electroretinogram in high intravitreal doses
   d severe periorbital skin rash and oedema
   e conjunctival cicatrization as a common adverse effect

8. **Retinal ganglion cells:**

   a transmit impulses faster in narrow-diameter axons
   b mediate the transmission of spatially coded signals
   c mostly have axons that contribute to the parvocellular system
   d that form the magnocellular system encode non-colour information
   e that form the parvocellular system encode high spatial frequency information

9. **Crystallins within the lens:**

   a may accumulate as high-molecular-weight aggregates, increasing transparency
   b include α crystallins which are present within the nucleus in young people
   c are important in maintaining transparency
   d constitute 20% of the total protein content of the lens
   e such as α crystallin are found in all lens cells

10. **Genetic and acquired defects in DNA include:**

   a transversions (conversion of a purine to another purine)
   b transitions, which are commoner than transversions
   c nonsense mutations, where splice sites are mutated
   d frameshift mutations, when base(s) are inserted or deleted from introns
   e deletions which involve relatively large segments of DNA (e.g. more than 40 base pairs)

11. **In Horner's syndrome:**

   a cocaine prevents reuptake of noradrenaline at adrenergic synapses
   b hydroxyamphetamine dilates a postganglionic sympathetic lesion
   c postganglionic lesions dilate with 1:1000 adrenaline
   d postganglionic lesions demonstrate denervation hypersensitivity
   e preganglionic and central lesions may be distinguished pharmacologically

12. **In Adie's pupil:**

   a light reactions are normal but the pupil remains dilated relative to the other eye
   b light reactions are normal but the near response is abolished
   c the defect results from damage to the ciliary ganglion
   d patients may present with blurred vision for near
   e physostigmine further dilates the pupil and this is used as a pharmacological aid in diagnosis

13. Mucosal associated lymphoid tissue:

a represents subepithelial accumulations of lymphoid tissue
b occurs as diffuse collections of lymphocytes, phagocytes, and plasma cells
c is present in the lung, gut, and appendix
d contains cells committed to IgA or IgE synthesis
e is constrained by a limiting capsular membrane

14. The following HLA types and diseases are associated:

a Behçet's and B27
b insulin dependent diabetes and B7
c multiple sclerosis and DR2
d sympathetic ophthalmia and A11
e Reiter's syndrome and B27

15. In X-linked dominant inheritance:

a the child of an affected mother is more likely to be affected than not
b affected children of an affected mother can be of either sex
c male-to-male transmission usually does not occur
d affected children of an affected father may be male
e Christmas disease is a prototype

16. Conjunctival tissue:

a is innervated inferiorly by branches of the maxillary division of the fifth cranial nerve
b receives parasympathetic nerve supply from the pterygopalatine ganglion
c is drained medially by submandibular lymph nodes
d is drained laterally by preauricular nodes
e epithelium forms a columnar multilayer in the fornices

17. Cranial neural crest gives rise to:

a extraocular muscle fibres
b neurosensory retina
c cartilage
d uveal melanocytes
e meningeal sheaths

18. The Golgi apparatus:

a contains membranes similar to the plasma membrane
b contains bound ribosomes within stacks of flattened lamellae
c interacts with rough endoplasmic reticulum
d contains mRNA for protein synthesis
e plays a major role in interacting with smooth endoplasmic reticulum

19. Complement activation:

a is regulated at one key rate-limiting step
b is regulated by complement receptors
c occurs via the lectin-activated alternative pathway
d may be triggered by free immunoglobulin
e induces the formation of the ion-permeable membrane attack complex

20. Media required for incubating micro-organisms include:

a thioglycolate broth for anaerobic bacteria only
b chocolate agar for *Neisseria* and *Haemophilus* species
c Thayer–Martin for *Neisseria meningitidis*
d Sabouraud for actinomycete infection
e Lowenstein–Jensen for non-tuberculous mycobacterial infection

21. The flash electroretinogram:

a typically presents light to the central 30 degrees of retina with Ganzfeld stimulation
b is larger in the dark-adapted eye
c may be recorded from an eyelid skin electrode
d features a positive polarity 'a' wave
e features a 'b' wave generated by outer retinal elements

22. Benzalkonium chloride:

    a is a surfactant preservative
    b is most effective at pH 6
    c causes papillary conjunctivitis
    d decreases bacterial cell wall permeability
    e is inactivated by calcium

23. The following enzyme(s) are abundant in the Golgi apparatus:

    a HMG-CoA reductase
    b glucose-6-phosphatase
    c HMG CoA
    d cytochrome P_{450}
    e sialyl transferase

24. With respect to immunoglobulin subclasses:

    a IgG is the predominant antibody in blood and lymph
    b IgA exists in dimeric form with the 'J' polypeptide link
    c IgD is present on the surface of many developing lymphocytes
    d IgM is found in breast milk
    e IgE is present on the surface of basophils

25. Thiazide diuretics:

    a are passively excreted into the proximal convoluted tubule
    b inhibit sodium ion reabsorption in the distal convoluted tubule
    c may decrease glomerular filtration
    d reduce urine pH
    e weakly inhibit carbonic anhydrase

26. Ciliary body epithelium:

    a produces aqueous humour at a rate of about 0.1 ml per hour
    b regulates intraocular pressure via adrenergic receptors
    c is the major site of action for pilocarpine (in reducing intraocular pressure)
    d contains more α_1 than α_2 adrenergic receptors
    e contains more β_1 than β_2 adrenergic receptors

27. **The following are parametric tests:**

    a Student t-test
    b chi-square test
    c analysis of variance
    d Fisher Exact test
    e Wilcoxon rank sum test

28. **Nonsteroidal anti-inflammatory agents such as aspirin:**

    a inhibit prostaglandin synthesis by inhibiting lipoxygenase
    b are rapidly metabolized by plasma esterases
    c are conjugated in the liver
    d may exacerbate gout
    e in overdose are treated with flumazenil

29. **In lymph nodes:**

    a B cells are present in primary and secondary nodules
    b T cells are present in deep tertiary cortex
    c secondary nodules lack macrophages
    d reticular fibres are found
    e B and T cells may proliferate

30. **Features of macrophages include:**

    a few microfilaments
    b few surface projections
    c many lysosomes
    d a round nucleus
    e active pinocytosis

31. **Interleukin 1:**

    a promotes leucocyte adhesion to endothelium
    b activates lymphocytes
    c is an endogenous pyrogen
    d induces fibroblast proliferation
    e is produced by endothelial cells

32. **The normal corneal endothelium:**

    a comprises 15 000 cells/mm² at birth
    b continues to replicate throughout life
    c is essential in maintaining corneal clarity by increasing corneal thickness
    d initially contains a heterogeneous cell population in terms of size
    e requires at least 1500 cells per mm² to function adequately

33. **The lacrimal gland:**

    a contains acini consisting of cylindrical eosinophilic secretory cells
    b is supplied by the lacrimal artery, a branch of the ophthalmic artery
    c receives a sympathetic nerve supply which synapses in the pterygopalatine ganglion
    d contains a larger palpebral portion
    e receives sympathetic supply via the lesser petrosal nerve

34. **The tear film:**

    a is 98% water
    b is slightly acidic
    c contains potassium at lower levels than in serum
    d contains amylase
    e contains retinol

35. **Delayed type IV hypersensitivity:**

    a requires T lymphocytes
    b is predominantly a humoral response
    c results in a mononuclear cell infiltration
    d is mediated by IgE antibodies bound to mast cells
    e is characterized by immune complex deposition

36. Tetracyclines:

a are bacteriostatic
b bind to the 50s subunit of the microbial ribosome, which leads to misreading of RNA code
c are well absorbed orally
d may damage developing teeth and bones
e are predominantly excreted by the kidney

37. Vitamin A:

a is hydrophobic and fat soluble
b is obtained from diet by beta carotene
c is incorporated into chylomicrons as a precursor of vitamin A and then released from the liver
d is carried in the bloodstream by retinol binding protein
e in excess increases gluconeogenesis and protein turnover

38. The following drugs act at the postsynaptic motor endplate:

a nicotine
b botulinum toxin
c neomycin
d hemicholinium
e latrotoxin

39. The iris:

a remains unformed as late as 3 months
b arises from neuroepithelial cells
c sphincter fibres develop first
d is formed by contributions from adrenergic and cholinergic fibres
e is nearly fully pigmented at term

40. Cerebrospinal fluid:

a usually contains a relatively high protein concentration
b has a lower calcium concentration than plasma
c has a lower glucose concentration than plasma
d has a greater pH than blood
e is an ultrafiltrate of plasma

41. Neutrophil granulocytes:

a are the commonest type of leucocyte in normal blood
b may increase in response to high levels of circulating glucocorticoids
c are reduced in number by drugs suppressing the bone marrow
d contain proteolytic enzymes
e have a life span of about 4 weeks

42. Blockade of parasympathetic activity causes an increase in:

a resting heart rate
b sweating
c salivation
d skeletal muscle contraction
e pupil diameter

43. The vitreous gel:

a absorbs 10% of visible light
b is most firmly attached to retina at the ora serrata
c has a refractive index of 1.38
d is acellular
e contains type II collagen

44. Cells of the retinal pigment epithelium:

a increase in number with age
b form a double layer arranged in a hexagonal format
c contain melanin granules
d are taller and more frequent at the fovea
e are smaller in the periphery

45. The following peptides are synthesized by neurosecretory neurones (originating from the hypothalamus):

a adrenaline (epinephrine)
b somatostatin
c somatomedin
d acetylcholine
e growth hormone

46. Aqueous humour:

a forms a total volume of about 2 ml in the anterior chamber
b forms a total volume of about 1 ml in the posterior chamber
c has a refractive index of 1.336
d contains more sodium and chloride in the posterior chamber
e contains transforming growth factor β

47. Drugs that may increase intraocular pressure include:

a amphotericin
b brimonidine
c amitriptyline
d fluorometholone
e beclometasone

48. Local anaesthetics:

a such as lignocaine have a negative inotropic effect
b when causing adverse reaction, usually do so because of inadvertent intravascular injection
c often cause allergic reactions affecting the skin
d should be used with caution in patients with epilepsy
e adverse reactions are more common with amide anaesthetics

49. When light strikes a photoreceptor outer segment:

a rhodopsin is deactivated
b sodium ions enter the cell through ion channels
c ion flow leads to a reduced level of depolarization
d cGMP closes sodium channels
e calcium is ultimately released at the synapse

50. The ciliary body:

a forms the pars plicata posteriorly
b lines the potential suprachoroidal space
c has an inner pigmented epithelium equivalent to the retinal pigment epithelium
d is innervated via short ciliary nerves which contain postganglionic parasympathetic fibres
e secretes hyaluronic acid into the vitreous

51. Descemet's membrane:

a readily regenerates in response to injury
b links corneal stroma to the endothelium
c forms a folded layer in normal circumstances
d has a posterior banded layer
e grows throughout life

52. Antihistamine drugs:

a have both local anaesthetic and anticholinergic properties
b prevent release of histamine from mast cells
c bind to H_1 receptors in the central nervous system making them effective anti-emetic agents
d inhibit gastric acid secretion
e may cause dry mouth, cough, palpitations, and headache

53. The vitreous cavity:

a contains sodium and potassium in similar concentrations to plasma
b contains a variety of different glycosaminoglycans in equal quantities
c contains hyaluronic acid, which is the major glycosaminoglycan
d contains collagen, which is the major structural protein
e contains low levels of ascorbic acid relative to plasma

54. Vertical nystagmus:

a may occur with phenytoin
b if downbeating, the lesion is usually in the midbrain
c is associated with oscillopsia
d if present in coma suggests poor hemispheric function
e may be caused by the Arnold–Chiari malformation

55. **The following are components of the electroretinogram:**

    a PIII
    b early receptor potential
    c oscillatory potential
    d a1 response
    e 'c' wave

56. **The polymerase chain reaction:**

    a depends on the synthesis of DNA by DNA polymerase
    b does not necessarily require pure DNA
    c requires equimolar concentrations of all four deoxynucleotide triphosphates
    d requires synthetic primers to anneal DNA and terminate synthesis
    e in the amplification phase is driven entirely by temperature change

57. **Class II major histocompatibility complex molecules:**

    a link to β_2 microglobulin
    b are transmembrane glycoproteins
    c contain α helices
    d contain β pleated sheets
    e form a heterodimer

58. **The following antibiotics inhibit cell wall synthesis:**

    a cefuroxime
    b vancomycin
    c sulphonamides
    d benzylpenicillin
    e erythromycin

59. **Advantages of sterilization by autoclave include:**

    a short sterilization time
    b reliability
    c the ability to clean rubber tubing in dry heat
    d the ability to kill resistant spores within 12 minutes
    e the ability to clean surgical instruments

60. Cytokine mediators:

    a are hormone-like lipoproteins
    b usually act as immunosuppressants
    c such as interferon-γ may induce MHC class II antigen expression
    d such as interleukin-3 are specifically lymphoproliferative
    e are secreted differentially by T cell subsets

Paper 3 – Questions

QUESTIONS

1. **The ciliary ganglion:**

   a receives two roots
   b has one short root derived from the nerve to the inferior oblique
   c contains sympathetic synapses
   d contains second order parasympathetic nerve cell bodies
   e gives rise to short ciliary nerves, which pierce the sclera around the optic nerve

2. **Regarding features of the cornea:**

   a type I and type III collagen are predominant within the stroma
   b Bowman's layer is a basement membrane
   c Bowman's layer is acellular
   d endothelial cells derive from neural crest
   e stroma is linked to Desçemet's membrane by collagen

3. **The lacrimal gland:**

   a measures approximately 2 cm by 3 cm by 1 cm
   b on its inferior surface is adjacent to the tendons of levator palpebrae superioris
   c contains a large palpebral portion
   d is usually visible when the upper lid is everted
   e is divided into its two portions by the aponeurosis of levator palpebrae superioris

4. **The optic tracts:**

   a receive a blood supply from the anterior choroidal artery
   b wind around the cerebral peduncles of the rostral midbrain
   c form a lateral root which terminates in the lateral geniculate nucleus
   d surround the third ventricle
   e lie above the posterior cerebral artery

5. **Streptococcus pneumoniae:**

    a   is a common cause of endocarditis
    b   is capsulated and sensitive to optochin
    c   ferments inulin
    d   causes lobar pneumonia
    e   is β haemolytic

6. **The contents of the anterior triangle of the neck include:**

    a   strap muscles
    b   the common carotid artery
    c   the carotid sinus and body
    d   the third part of the subclavian artery
    e   the inferior belly of omohyoid

7. **Neural crest:**

    a   chick–quail chimeras help trace neural crest development
    b   forms the trabecular meshwork
    c   forms the corneal epithelium
    d   forms part of the sclera
    e   arises from the forebrain

8. **Concerning the development of the face:**

    a   it starts around week 4
    b   it is largely completed by week 10
    c   the nasolacrimal groove is formed by fusion of the maxillary process with the medial nasal swelling
    d   vitamin A deficiency is associated with anophthalmia
    e   the upper and lower eyelids are initially fused

9. **Concerning the development of the cornea:**

    a   the first wave of mesenchyme forms corneal stroma
    b   the first wave of mesenchyme forms corneal endothelium
    c   wing cells are the first cells to appear in the epithelium
    d   collagen bundles mature into a regular array anteriorly first
    e   keratoblasts appear during the first trimester

10. **The following are derived from the 2nd pharyngeal arch:**

    a   epithelial lining of the tonsils
    b   Reichert's cartilage
    c   stapes bone
    d   part of parathyroid gland
    e   part of hyoid bone

11. **Development of vitreous:**

    a   starts at 12 weeks with the formation of primary vitreous
    b   initially is probably derived from ectoderm and mesoderm
    c   in the secondary phase has a prominent vascular component
    d   in the tertiary stage forms the vitreous base
    e   is formed by each section of the trilaminar disk

12. **Regarding the development of the optic nerve:**

    a   the optic stalk starts to close over the hyaloid vessels at 5–6 weeks
    b   the choroidal fissure is closed by 6 weeks' gestation
    c   Bergmeister's papilla represents nerve tissue at the disk
    d   the optic nerve is displaced nasally with temporal zone expansion
    e   malformed lamina cribrosa causes Morning Glory syndrome

13. **The superior oblique muscle:**

    a   acts at an angle of 23 degrees
    b   arises from the sphenoid bone lateral to the optic foramen
    c   only depresses the globe in adduction
    d   is supplied by the fourth cranial nerve on its lower surface
    e   intorts the globe from the primary position

14. **Regarding the pharyngeal arches:**

    a arch 3 forms the upper part of the hyoid bone
    b arch 1 forms the anterior belly of digastric
    c arch 4 forms the superior parathyroid
    d arch 4 forms the upper laryngeal cartilages
    e arch 1 forms the tympanic cavity

15. **Eosinophil polymorphonuclear leucocytes are present in:**

    a cat scratch disease
    b vernal conjunctivitis
    c pulmonary eosinophilia
    d juvenile xanthogranuloma
    e tuberculous conjunctivitis

16. **Deposition of elastic tissue is a feature of:**

    a syphilitic aortitis
    b pterygium
    c intimal proliferation in muscular arteries
    d actinic keratosis
    e rheumatoid arthritis

17. **Pigmentation of tissues follows:**

    a haemorrhage
    b application of silver nitrate solution
    c topical application of adrenaline derivatives
    d destruction of the adrenals
    e application of topical steroids

18. **The following cells are known to exhibit reactionary proliferation:**

    a choroidal melanocytes
    b retinal pigment epithelium
    c conjunctival lymphocytes
    d corneal endothelial cells
    e corneal stromal cells

19. **The following systemic diseases can cause intraocular inflammation:**

    a Behçet's disease
    b syphilis
    c sarcoidosis
    d systemic lupus erythematosus
    e subacute bacterial endocarditis

20. **Multinucleate giant cells occur in response to the following infections:**

    a tuberculosis
    b candidiasis
    c herpes zoster
    d acanthamoebal keratitis
    e actinomycosis

21. **Metastatic calcification occurs in:**

    a hypoparathyroidism
    b sarcoidosis
    c uveitis
    d hypervitaminosis D
    e hyperthyroidism

22. **Lymphocytic infiltration is a feature of:**

    a organizing haemorrhage in the vitreous
    b extraocular muscle in thyroid eye disease
    c vitreous abscess
    d the optic nerve in multiple sclerosis
    e the lacrimal gland in Sjögren's syndrome

23. **Tumours derived from epithelial cells can be characterized by:**

    a desmosomal attachments
    b the presence of cytokeratins
    c intracytoplasmic immunoglobulins
    d neurosecretory granules
    e mucin granules

24. The external carotid artery:

a lies superficial to the facial nerve within the parotid gland
b forms the maxillary artery as a single terminal continuation
c does not anastamose with the internal carotid circulation
d gives rise to the facial artery below the lingual artery
e lies lateral to the internal carotid artery at its origin

25. Melanin pigmentation is observed in:

a basal cell carcinoma
b basal cell papilloma
c compound naevus
d Merkel cell carcinoma
e sebaceous adenoma

26. Malignant soft tissue tumours:

a always occur in elderly patients
b occur more frequently in patients with a 13q/14 deletion
c metastasize via lymphatics
d metastasize to lungs
e are identified by cytokeratin markers

27. In temporal arteritis a biopsy may reveal:

a intimal fibroplasia
b multinucleate cells in the region of the internal elastic layer
c calcification of the internal elastic layer
d lymphocytes around the adventitial vessels
e an organizing thrombus in the lumen

28. In which of the following diseases is a necrotizing vasculitis a feature?

a diabetes
b Takayasu's disease
c Wegener's granulomatosis
d systemic lupus erythematosus
e medionecrosis of the aorta (dissecting aneurysm)

29. **The optic chiasm may be compressed by:**

    a   a pinealoma
    b   a craniopharyngioma
    c   a pituitary adenoma
    d   an aneurysm on the basilar artery
    e   a pontine glioma

30. **Birefringent crystals are seen in the tissues in:**

    a   gout
    b   cystinosis
    c   lipid keratopathy
    d   asteroid hyalosis
    e   homocystinuria

31. **Photoreceptor atrophy is a feature of:**

    a   central retinal vein occlusion
    b   retinal detachment
    c   retinitis pigmentosa
    d   sclerosis of choroidal vessels
    e   Tay–Sachs disease

32. **The nerve fibre layer of the retina is atrophic in:**

    a   central retinal artery occlusion
    b   glaucoma
    c   retinal detachment
    d   diabetic retinopathy
    e   Tay–Sachs disease

33. **In corneal development:**

    a   the endothelium forms a single layer at week 6
    b   collagen fibres can be detected by the third month
    c   Descemet's membrane is formed last
    d   the first wave of neural crest cell migration forms iris
         and pupillary membrane
    e   keratocytes form initially in the posterior cornea

34. Landmarks in retinal development include:

a synaptogenesis in rods before cones
b outer segment formation at about 5 months
c horizontal cell formation around the 5th month
d the transient layer of Chievitz at 2 months
e centripetal differentiation from the retinal periphery

35. Features of the lateral wall of the orbit include:

a a lateral orbital tubercle which is the origin of the check ligament of the lateral rectus
b spina recti lateralis which gives origin to part of the superior rectus
c foramina for small veins that communicate with the middle cranial fossa
d the zygomatic foramen which transmits only the zygomatic nerve
e the greater wing of the sphenoid

36. Herpes viruses:

a are RNA viruses
b can be distinguished by electron microscopy
c may cross the placenta
d are associated with malignancy
e are latent viruses

37. Actinomycosis infection:

a may be disseminated
b is best treated with benzylpenicillin
c most commonly affects the lung
d spreads via the lymphatics
e typically leads to giant cell formation

38. β haemolytic streptococci:

a all possess Lancefield group B antigen
b cause erysipelas and impetigo
c contain M protein in the cell wall
d are associated with post-infectious glomerulonephritis
e may cause neonatal septicaemia and pneumonia

39. ***Cytomegalovirus*** **infection:**

   a is the commonest eye infection in acquired immunodeficiency syndrome
   b causes large cytoplasmic inclusions
   c may reactivate in renal transplant patients
   d grows readily in cell culture
   e stimulates giant cell production

40. **Recognized features of toxoplasmosis include:**

   a transmission from cats and sheep
   b a predilection for immunocompromised patients
   c congenital chorioretinitis and cerebral palsy
   d peripheral blood monocytosis
   e thrombocytopenia

41. ***Chlamydia trachomatis*:**

   a cannot grow alone
   b divide by binary fission
   c grow in cell culture (McCoy media)
   d are intracellular
   e are sensitive to penicillin

42. **Meningococcal infection:**

   a is caused by Gram-positive diplococci
   b may cause endophthalmitis without meningitis
   c is penicillin sensitive
   d has steadily increased in incidence over the last decade
   e is caused by oxidase-negative bacteria

43. **Concerning the development of the skull:**

   a the first pharyngeal arch forms the upper jaw
   b the second pharyngeal arch forms the lower jaw
   c each arch has an inner covering of ectoderm
   d the maxillary bone condenses from neural crest
   e Treacher Collins syndrome represents a defect in neural crest development

44. In lens development:

a   induction of primary lens fibres occurs at about day 49
b   the tunica vasculosa lentis forms an essential function
c   secondary lens fibres arise from the posterior epithelium
d   the tunica vasculosa lentis encloses the lens by week 6
e   the lens cavity transiently connects with the amniotic cavity

45. Sclera:

a   is reinforced around rectus muscle insertions
b   is derived from mesenchyme
c   forms three well-defined layers
d   is thinnest beneath the recti
e   contains collagen, predominantly type II

46. *Staphylococcus aureus*:

a   is catalase positive
b   is coagulase positive
c   may cause toxic shock syndrome
d   is carried by at least 30% of a normal population
e   ferments mannitol

47. The anterior lamella of the upper lid:

a   contains Müller's muscle, which acts to elevate the lid
b   contains orbicularis oculi fibres
c   features the ciliary glands of Moll
d   offers the most structural support to the lid
e   contains modified hair follicles with arrector pili muscle

48. The ophthalmic artery:

a   is a terminal branch of the external carotid artery
b   arises at source within the cavernous sinus
c   lies medial to the optic nerve in the optic canal
d   forms the ophthalmic artery, which is an end-artery
e   arises in the middle cranial fossa, lateral to the anterior clinoid process

49. *Staphylococcus aureus*:

a usually causes fever
b is catalase positive
c is coagulase negative
d ferments mannitol
e is β haemolytic

50. DNA viruses:

a usually contain single-stranded DNA
b have a helical structure
c usually contain circular DNA
d include adenovirus and hepatitis A viruses
e replicate in the cytoplasm

51. Features of the floor of the middle cranial fossa include:

a the optic canal between the crista galli and the lesser wing of the sphenoid
b the superior orbital fissure, which lies at the apex of the cavernous sinus
c the foramen rotundum, which transmits the mandibular nerve
d the foramen lacerum at the apex of the petrous temporal bone
e the foramen spinosum, which lies anterior to the foramen ovale

52. The following pass through the foramen magnum:

a pons
b basilar artery
c vertebral artery
d posterior vertebral venous plexus
e the carotid rootlets of the upper cervical nerves

53. Gonococcal infection:

a is caused by Gram-negative microaerophilic diplococci, which may be grown on chocolate agar plates
b only rarely causes eye problems
c is usually transmitted via the bloodstream to the eye
d is not naturally found in humans
e leads to pseudomembrane formation

54. The choroid:

a is formed from mesenchyme surrounding the optic cup
b arises very early in eye development (at about 2 months)
c forms four primitive layers during its development
d contains pigment-bearing melanocytes around month 3
e forms the fenestrated choriocapillaris from venous channels

55. In the 10-week-old embryo:

a the approximate length of the embryo is 2 cm
b tarsal glands are undeveloped
c ciliary muscle is formed
d optic nerve myelination begins
e retinal differentiation begins

56. Mesoderm derivatives include:

a orbital walls
b extraocular muscles
c Tenon's capsule
d sclera and choroid
e Desçemet's membrane

57. The following are derived from the 2nd pharyngeal arch:

a thyroid cartilage
b incus bone
c stapes bone
d malleus bone
e stylopharyngeus

58. Corneal stroma:

a predominantly contains type II collagen
b accounts for 90% of corneal thickness
c contains numerous axons and Schwann cells in its posterior third
d consists of lamellae which extend from limbus to limbus
e is maintained by keratocytes, which constantly produce collagen and extracellular matrix

59. Onchocerciasis:

a causes 'river blindness'
b is endemic in the river basins of West and Central Africa
c is caused by microfilaria which reach the anterior surface of the eye via the bloodstream
d provides an example of molecular mimicry
e is transmitted from the black fly to humans and humans may reinfect the black fly

60. Lipopolysaccharide:

a causes fever and hypotension
b contains lipid A
c contains core polysaccharide which is mainly responsible for its systemic effects
d activates complement
e causes neutropenia

Paper 4 – Questions

QUESTIONS

1. **Restriction endonuclease enzymes:**

   a are used in Southern blotting
   b are used to identify DNA polymorphisms
   c are used in the polymerase chain reaction
   d are used for gene mapping
   e with DNA ligase are used to incorporate DNA sequences into plasmids

2. **Characteristic features of Turner's syndrome include:**

   a tall stature
   b short neck and low hairline
   c aortic stenosis
   d cubitus valgus
   e ovarian dysgenesis

3. **Autosomal dominant conditions include:**

   a Stickler's syndrome
   b tritanopia
   c Best's disease
   d familial ectopia lentis
   e macular corneal dystrophy

4. **The following diseases are autosomal recessive:**

   a Meesman's corneal dystrophy
   b hexosaminidase A deficiency
   c simple myopia
   d Stargardt's dystrophy
   e retinoblastoma

5. **Mitochondrial DNA:**

   a contains universal code throughout
   b is exclusively paternally derived
   c is present in sperm
   d is double stranded and linear
   e codes for tRNA proteins

6. **The cornea is transparent because:**

   a of the regular arrangement of stromal type II collagen

   b Bowman's layer contains a regular layer of collagen fibrils

   c collagen fibrils in the cornea are mostly of uniform thickness

   d type III collagen creates a lattice arrangement

   e glycosaminoglycans are hydrophobic

7. **Concerning the mechanisms of colour vision:**

   a the opponent theory can be explained at the ganglion cell level

   b trichromatic and opponent theories are mutually exclusive

   c they are subserved by the magnocellular pathway

   d there is good evidence for three types of cones

   e the V4 region in the occipital cortex plays an important role

8. **Regarding electrolytes in the cornea:**

   a sodium is present in relatively high concentrations in the stroma

   b sodium is partly regulated by bicarbonate-regulated ATPase

   c the epithelial potassium concentration is about ~ 5 mmol/l

   d Na$^+$/K$^+$ ATPase is found on the endothelial layer

   e carbonic anhydrase is thought to regulate sodium and bicarbonate transport

9. **Recognized features of trisomy 13 (Patau syndrome) include:**

   a malformed cornea and chamber angle

   b persistent hyperplastic primary vitreous

   c retinal dysplasia

   d optic nerve hypoplasia

   e anterior coloboma

10. **The antibiotic vancomycin:**

   a is primarily effective against facultative Gram-negative rods
   b is not recommended for routine use in ocular irrigation fluids to prevent endophthalmitis
   c is very poorly absorbed when taken orally
   d inhibits protein and cell wall synthesis
   e is excreted by the kidneys

11. **Bruch's membrane:**

   a separates the basal surface of the retinal pigment epithelium from the choriocapillaris
   b has an inner layer composed mainly of collagen
   c contains basement membrane and an inner and outer collagen zone
   d serves as a barrier to macromolecules passing from choriocapillaris to retinal pigment epithelium
   e remains of constant thickness with age

12. **Müller cells:**

   a are glial cells
   b provide retina with nutrition
   c have a basement membrane which forms the inner limiting membrane of the retina
   d produce the 'b' wave of the electroretinogram
   e produce the 'a' wave of the electroretinogram

13. **Over 120 million rods and 6 millions cones form the neurosensory retina. Which of the following statements is/are correct?:**

   a rod density increases with distance from the macula up to the extreme periphery
   b rods are recycled on a daily basis
   c cone density is approximately 6000/mm^2 in the periphery
   d rod density is greatest in the superonasal retina
   e rod density is high at the fovea

14. **Mydriatic agents with cycloplegic action include:**

    a cyclopentolate
    b atropine
    c phenylephrine
    d homatropine
    e physostigmine

15. **The vital capacity of the lungs:**

    a equates to the expiratory reserve volume added to the inspiratory capacity
    b is the maximal volume of gas that can be expired after a maximal inspiration
    c is the sum of the tidal volume and the inspiratory reserve volume
    d is the sum of the functional residual capacity and inspiratory capacity
    e is virtually the same as the total lung capacity

16. **The null hypothesis:**

    a is rejected when it is true in type I error
    b is accepted when the alternative hypothesis is false in type II error
    c usually proposes that the trial assertion is false
    d is rejected with a P value of 0.06
    e if proven provides evidence for the alternative hypothesis

17. **Mitochondria perform the following function(s):**

    a steroid synthesis
    b ATP synthesis
    c polysaccharide breakdown
    d electron transport
    e DNA synthesis

18. **The intracellular matrix:**

    a contains microfilaments which are coiled α helices
    b features mesenchymal vimentin intermediate filaments
    c is deformable because of actin microfilaments
    d contains desmin, which interconnects myofibrils
    e contains lipofuscin in RPE cells

19. **Retinal pigment epithelial cells:**

    a contain melanosomes and lysosomes
    b recycle 11-*cis* retinal and store retinoid unbound in cytoplasm
    c produce the 'a' wave of the electroretinogram
    d utilize the P_{450} drug-metabolizing system
    e secrete interleukin-1

20. **The visual evoked potential:**

    a is recorded with scalp electrodes
    b is derived predominantly from peripheral retina
    c may be recorded using a high-contrast reversing chequerboard
    d measures the response of the entire retina
    e is generated using a cathode ray tube screen that subtends 10–15° of visual angle

21. **Antigen presentation:**

    a is usually performed by dendritic cells
    b is a process that allows macrophages to release interleukin-1
    c requires MHC class II molecules
    d to T cells is effective without antigen processing
    e may result in T cell death

22. **Endotoxins:**

    a activate complement
    b may be secreted by Gram-positive bacteria
    c readily induce a protective antibody response
    d are lipopolysaccharides
    e contain lipid A

23. **Human housekeeping genes:**

    a control the basal metabolic activity of a cell
    b usually display variable expression
    c that code for ubiquitin play a key role in protein synthesis
    d that code for phospholipase A_2 are involved with lipid metabolism
    e include the major histocompatibility complex

24. Stimulation of renin secretion:

a increases serum potassium concentrations
b increases extracellular fluid volume
c decreases plasma colloid oncotic pressure
d decreases serum sodium concentrations
e leads to angiotensinogen formation

25. Non-parametric statistical tests are used to:

a analyse non-categorical data
b analyse unequal group sizes with the unpaired t test
c analyse small sample sizes ($n<5$) with the chi-square test
d correlate using a ranking system to calculate probability values
e analyse regression of normally distributed data

26. Glycogen synthesis:

a occurs in the well-fed state
b requires an activated form of glucose, glucose-1-phosphate
c is promoted by insulin
d requires uridine triphosphate
e requires glucokinase

27. Glucose transport by insulin-dependent facilitated diffusion occurs in:

a adipose tissue
b cardiac muscle
c skeletal muscle
d the central nervous system
e the kidney

28. Collagen type I:

a is abundant in skin and bone
b is the predominant form of collagen in basement membranes surrounding smooth muscle cells
c contains three identical $\alpha_1$chains wound into a superhelix
d is the predominant form of collagen in basement membranes
e is the predominant form of collagen in cartilage and the vitreous body

29. Varicella zoster virus:

a   is associated with human cancer
b   is a double-stranded RNA virus
c   may infect both sensory ganglia and motor nerves
d   is associated with eosinophilic nuclear inclusion bodies
e   occasionally causes shingles as a primary infection

30. The pattern electroretinogram:

a   operates by default at 50 Hz
b   produces a signal amplitude of 100 mV
c   is generated predominantly by the lateral geniculate nuclei
d   is reduced in complete optic nerve section
e   requires signal averaging

31. The neurohypophysis contains the following cell types:

a   gonadotrophs
b   chromophobes
c   acidophils
d   basophils
e   lactotropes

32. With respect to Horner's syndrome:

a   phenylephrine dilates the pupils equally in
    preganglionic lesions
b   there is variable loss of sweating over the affected side
    of the face
c   it may occur in the lateral medullary syndrome
d   it may follow damage to the lower trunks of the
    brachial plexus
e   hydroxyamphetamine drops dilate the pupil if the
    lesion is postganglionic

33. In type II hypersensitivity:

a   antigen is not necessarily present on the cell surface
b   complement is a key component
c   cell-mediated cytotoxicity may be mediated by polymorphs
d   cell-mediated cytotoxicity may be mediated by monocytes
e   complement produces direct membrane damage

34. **Autosomal dominant conditions:**

   a are usually more severe than autosomal recessive disorders
   b include myotonic dystrophy
   c include Marfan's syndrome
   d include homocystinuria and Weil–Marchesani syndrome
   e include complete colour blindness

35. **Concerning rhodopsin:**

   a it binds vitamin A
   b it is an external cell membrane protein
   c opsin is a seven-turn α helix
   d it behaves like a receptor
   e it is activated by isomerization of retinal

36. **Angle-closure glaucoma may be in part precipitated by:**

   a tropicamide more than cyclopentolate
   b antimuscarinic agents
   c topical β blockers
   d atropine
   e tricyclic antidepressants

37. **T lymphocytes produce the following cytokines:**

   a interleukin-1
   b interleukin-2
   c interleukin-3
   d TNF-α
   e interleukin-4

38. **Complement activation is regulated by:**

   a inhibitors for surface-bound complement
   b serine protease inhibitors
   c universal cell surface proteins such as vitronectin
   d a collection of nine α globulins
   e red cell lysis

39. **With respect to epithelial cell turnover:**

    a it depends on the viability of limbal epithelial cell
       population
    b stem cells divide to self-renew and to form terminally
       differentiated cells
    c regenerating cells are less likely to stimulate
       vascularization
    d corneal epithelium can completely regenerate within
       1–2 days
    e hemidesmosomes form within 18 hours following
       corneal abrasion

40. **Class I major histocompatibility complex molecules:**

    a are transmembrane glycoproteins
    b consist of covalently linked peptide chains
    c contain α helices
    d contain β pleated sheets
    e form a heterodimer

41. **In X linked recessive conditions:**

    a a heterozygous female with Turner's syndrome will not
       be affected
    b usually only males are affected
    c phenotypically normal daughters of affected males are
       not carriers
    d Aicardi syndrome is a prototype
    e an affected male transmits the gene to all daughters
       and none of his sons

42. **The corneal stroma:**

    a consists of about 20 collagen lamellae oriented at 90° to
       each other
    b drains waste products via lymph channels
    c accounts for 90% of corneal thickness
    d is formed by lamellae, each about 100 μm thick
    e contains fibres which blend directly with scleral
       collagen

43. The otic ganglion:

a is located above the foramen ovale
b is located medial to the inferior maxillary nerve
c is anterior to the middle meningeal artery
d distributes branches to tensor palati and tensor tympani
e lies at the level of the origin of the maxillary division of the fifth cranial nerve

44. Intraocular pressure:

a varies 1–2 mm with inspiration
b is highest in the evening
c is measured by applanation (Imbert–Fick principle)
d is underestimated with a Schiotz (indentation) tonometer if scleral rigidity is low (e.g. in myopia)
e is underestimated in higher ranges by the non-contact tonometer

45. Acetazolamide:

a inhibits an enzyme that uses water as a substrate
b causes sodium retention
c decreases aqueous outflow
d causes hyperchloraemic metabolic acidosis
e causes hyperkalaemia

46. Human insulin:

a has a plasma half life of 30 minutes
b may be formed from pork insulin by substituting one amino acid
c is longer-acting in soluble form
d is longer-acting when combined with protamine
e is constructed from three polypeptide chains

47. Warfarin:

a inactivates vitamin K
b leads to the production of inactive clotting factors
c takes 4 days to take effect
d is 99% bound to plasma albumin
e metabolism is stimulated by chloramphenicol

48. β-**adrenoceptor blocking drugs:**

   a block β-adrenoceptors in the heart, peripheral vasculature, pancreas, and liver

   b like acebutolol have intrinsic sympathomimetic activity

   c like atenolol are lipid soluble

   d all slow the heart rate

   e must not be given in diabetics with a tendency to hypoglycaemia

49. Mast cells:

   a exist in two forms

   b have a low affinity for IgE Fc

   c bind IgE molecules, which crosslink, thus triggering mediator release

   d contain phosphatidyl inositol

   e release preformed leukotriene B_4

50. Local anaesthetics:

   a inhibit potassium channels of the nerve membrane

   b contain a hydrophilic amino group

   c when combined with adrenaline (epinephrine) are less likely themselves to cause a systemic reaction

   d that contain adrenaline (epinephrine) have a shorter duration of action

   e such as bupivacaine have a relatively slow rate of onset of effect

51. Glucocorticoids:

   a inhibit gluconeogenesis

   b increase resistance to stress

   c increase the eosinophil count

   d lower the peripheral lymphocyte count

   e activate phospholipase A_2

52. Sulphonamides:

a are structurally related to *p*-aminobenzoic acid
b are effective because bacteria absorb folic acid
c interfere with amino acid synthesis
d interfere with purine and pyrimidine synthesis
e are effective against *Chlamydia*

53. The following substances are present in aqueous humour at higher concentrations than in plasma:

a glucose
b lactate
c ascorbate
d oxygen
e calcium

54. Platelet-derived growth factor:

a is mitogenic
b is found primarily within platelets, monocytes, and endothelial cells
c exists in monomeric form
d is implicated in tissue inflammation and repair after trauma
e is present in aqueous humour

55. Intraocular pressure typically increases with the following:

a age
b after consumption of 1 litre of water
c axial length
d administration of ketamine anaesthesia
e administration of suxamethonium

56. Confidence intervals:

a typically indicate the level of confidence at the 0.90 probability level
b are calculated from the mean and standard deviation
c depend on sample size
d if wide suggest that the sample size may be too small
e are wider when standard deviation is greater

57. Concerning red blood cell inclusions:

a when observed post-splenectomy are called Heinz bodies

b in glucose-6-phosphate deficiency are called Howell–Jolly bodies

c are basophilic in lead poisoning

d are found in siderocytes as iron deposits

e when composed of RNA are known as reticulocytes

58. Inhibitors of nucleic acid synthesis:

a such as aciclovir inhibit DNA polymerase and terminal chain elongation

b such as ganciclovir are 100 times more active against *Cytomegalovirus* than aciclovir

c are usually well absorbed orally

d are often nucleoside analogues that require phosphorylation to exert their antiviral effects

e such as amantadine are fraudulent bases

59. Chloramphenicol:

a attaches to the P site of microbial ribosomes and inhibits tRNA attachments

b is not effective in treating anaerobic or rickettsial infections

c penetrates well into cerebrospinal fluid owing to its high lipid solubility

d is excreted by the liver

e is associated with the 'grey baby syndrome'

60. Fluoroquinolone antibiotics:

a are chemically related to nalidixic acid

b inhibit DNA polymerase

c are usually bacteriostatic

d are especially useful in Gram-positive infections

e taken orally are not suitable for those under the age of 18

Paper 1 – Answers

ANSWERS

1. The oculomotor nerve

a True
b False
c True
d False
e False

The oculomotor nerve passes lateral to the posterior communicating artery. The parasympathetic fibres are the most superficial and they may be damaged first in intracranial injury. Cavernous sinus lesions more commonly affect oculomotor and trochlear nerves compared to the abducent nerve, which is protected by the internal carotid artery.

2. The superior orbital fissure

a True
b False
c True
d False
e False

The two divisions of the oculomotor nerve, the nasociliary nerve, and the abducent nerve pass within the common tendinous ring. The superior orbital fissure lies between the roof and the lateral wall of the orbit.

3. The corneal epithelium

a True
b False
c True
d True
e False

The corneal epithelium is about 50 μm thick, and is devoid of melanin and dendritic cells centrally. The glycocalyx is a layer of macromolecules that covers the external surface of the cell membrane. Glycocalyx glycoproteins are important in many cell recognition phenomena.

4. Staphylococcus aureus

a False
b True
c True
d True
e True

Staphylococcus aureus is carried nasally in 70–90% of the population, but only 30% are found to be persistent carriers. It causes about 30% of infective endocarditis.

5. Roundworm infestation

a True
b False
c True
d False
e True

Loiasis is transmitted by deer fly. Black fly is the intermediate host for onchocerciasis (and may be diagnosed by skin biopsy). Trichinella spiralis is a nematode parasite that lives in gut mucosa; human infection is usually the result of eating undercooked pork. Dogs are the natural hosts of Toxocara canis.

6. The cornea contains

a True
b False
c False
d True
e True

The cornea contains only a small amount of hyaluronic acid. The glycosaminoglycans are predominantly keratan sulphate and chondroitin sulphate. The corneal stroma normally contains no lymphatic or blood channels. Bowman's layer consists of randomly arranged collagen fibrils (types I, III, V, and VI).

7. The cavernous sinus

a True
b True

c **True**
d **True**
e **False**

The cavernous sinus also directly communicates with the superior petrosal sinus. The maxillary nerve travels in the inferolateral wall.

---

8. The right fourth nerve nucleus

a **False**
b **False**
c **True**
d **True**
e **True**

Even though this nerve is the smallest cranial nerve, it contains over 20 000 fibres. It originates ventral to the inferior colliculus in caudal midbrain. Each fourth cranial nerve is crossed, innervating the contralateral superior oblique.

---

9. Corneal endothelial cells

a **False**
b **True**
c **True**
d **False**
e **True**

The endothelium is a simple squamous epithelium that rests on Desçemet's membrane. There are about 4000 cells per square millimetre at birth. The lateral surfaces of endothelial cells are highly interdigitated (indicative of their crucial role in fluid transport).

---

10. The following are paired venous sinuses

a **True**
b **False**
c **True**
d **True**
e **False**

The dural venous sinuses are valveless, highly specialized, firm-walled veins within the cranial cavity, which drain venous blood from the brain. The solitary straight sinus joins the superior sagittal vein to form two transverse sinuses. The occipital sinuses lie on either side of foramen magnum. The bilateral petrosal sinuses drain from the cavernous sinuses to the sigmoid sinuses.

11. The sclera

a False
b True
c False
d False
e True

Sclera has a similar water content to cornea (approximately 70% and 80% respectively) but contains less than half the amount of glycosaminoglycans. Sclera is thickest posteriorly (1 mm) and thinnest (0.3–0.4 mm) below the insertions of the tendons of extraocular muscles. Sclera consists principally of collagen types I and III.

12. In ciliary body development

a False
b False
c True
d True
e False

Ciliary body (and iris) development starts at the eleventh to twelfth week, whereas the lens develops from about day 27. The *Hox* gene is a highly specialized marker of cells that subsequently form ciliary body and iris. The inner layer of the developing neuroectoderm is *non-pigmented*. Aqueous develops from week 20, as the trabecular meshwork drainage channels form.

13. The limbus

a False
b True
c True
d True
e ~~True~~ *false*

The limbus is 1.5–2.0 mm in width. Desçemet's membrane and Bowman's layer terminate in this region.

14. **Clostridium botulinum**

   a **True**
   b **True**
   c **False**
   d **False**
   e **False**

   Types A, B and E are the commonest serotypes which cause disease. Botulinum toxin-A acts by a contraction-dependent inhibition of release of acetylcholine from the motor nerve terminal.

15. **The optic nerve**

   a **False**
   b **False**
   c **True**
   d **False**
   e **True**

   The optic nerve consists of second order neurones. The optic nerve length varies from 35 to 55 mm, but averages 40 mm. Individual section lengths: intraocular 0.7 mm; intraorbital 3 cm; canalicular 6 mm; intracranial 1 cm.

16. **The lateral geniculate bodies**

   a **False**
   b **False**
   c **True**
   d **True**
   e **True**

   The lateral geniculate nuclei are part of the thalamus. Nerve fibres from the ipsilateral eye terminate in layers 2, 3, and 5.

17. **Bruch's membrane**

   a **False**
   b **False**

71

c   **True**
d   **True**
e   **True**

Bruch's membrane is a modified connective tissue layer, 2–4 μm thick and histologically appears as an acellular glassy membrane beneath the RPE.

---

18. **In the 6-week-old embryo**

a   **False**
b   **False**
c   **True**
d   **False**
e   **False**

The fetal fissure starts to close at this stage. The optic chiasm and secondary lens fibres form at 8 weeks. Myelination of the optic nerve begins at the optic chiasm at the fourth month of fetal life and reaches the lamina cribrosa at term.

---

19. **The following are derived from the 1st pharyngeal arch**

a   **True**
b   **False**
c   **False**
d   **False**
e   **False**

The greater horn of the hyoid bone forms from the 2nd arch. Stylopharyngeus forms from the 3rd arch. The upper laryngeal cartilages form from the 4th arch, the lower laryngeal cartilages from the 6th arch.

---

20. **Crystallins in lens cells**

a   **False**
b   **False**
c   **True**
d   **True**
e   **True**

Crystallins are water soluble; there are three types in mammals (α, β, and γ).

21. Concerning the iris

a True
b False
c False
d True
e False

The dilator muscle develops late (at about 6 months) and forms as an extension from the anterior epithelium. At about 13 weeks, anterior iris pigment epithelial cells lose their melanin. Aniridia is linked to chromosome 11 (short arm) not chromosome 17.

22. Components of the vitreous include

a True
b False
c True
d False
e True

Vitreous is formed by 98% water, with a refractive index of 1.33. Its main component is fine diameter type II collagen fibres which entrap hyaluronic acid molecules.

23. The orbital margin

a True
b False
c True
d False
e True

The margin is formed from the frontal, maxillary, lacrimal, and zygomatic bones, and is thickest and concave laterally.

24. The following structures form part of the midbrain

a True
b True
c False
d True
e True

The nucleus ambiguus is in the medulla.

---

25. **In diabetic microangiopathy**

    a True
    b True
    c True
    d False
    e False

    Hard exudates form in the outer plexiform layer. Micro-aneurysms contain PAS-positive material at a relatively late stage in their formation.

---

26. **The first division of the trigeminal nerve**

    a False
    b True
    c False
    d False
    e True

    The first division of the trigeminal nerve is the smallest, and divides into the lacrimal, frontal, and nasociliary branches. The lacrimal nerve enters the orbit above the annulus of Zinn.

---

27. **The meibomian glands**

    a True
    b False
    c False
    d True
    e False

    Meibomian glands form a single row in each lid. There are 20–30 glands in the lower lid and 30–40 in the upper lid.

---

28. **Branches of the internal carotid artery include**

    a True
    b True
    c True
    d True
    e False

The submaxillary artery is a branch of the external carotid artery.

---

29. **Metastases can occur in the following tissue layers**

    a True
    b True
    c True
    d True
    e False

---

30. **Dystrophic calcification can occur within**

    a True
    b True
    c False
    d True
    e True

---

31. **In various forms of embolic disease the pulmonary arterioles may contain**

    a True
    b True
    c False
    d False
    e True

---

32. **The following cells participate in allograft rejection**

    a False
    b True
    c True
    d False
    e False

    Allograft rejection may be hyperacute, acute or chronic. If, for example, no ABO mismatch has occurred inducing hyper- and acute rejection, chronic rejection is mediated by autoantigen presentation to $CD4^+$ and $CD8^+$ T cells. Graft rejection is thus markedly reduced with longterm immunosuppression.

33. **In a fracture in a bone it is possible to identify**

   a False
   b True
   c True
   d True
   e False

34. **In pathological states the following may be deposited in the extracellular matrix**

   a True
   b False
   c True
   d True
   e False

   Iron can be deposited in tissues and extracellular matrix during iron overload and haemochromatosis. Graves' disease increases glycosaminoglycans in orbital tissue and calcium is found in dystrophic and malignant states.

35. **The following tumours have the capacity to metastasize to distant sites**

   a True
   b False
   c True
   d True
   e False

36. **In ischaemia the following tissue components are identified**

   a False
   b True
   c False
   d True
   e True

37. **Irradiation therapy causes**

   a True
   b True
   c False

d False

e True

---

38. **Regarding features of pharyngeal arch development**

    a False
    b True
    c False
    d True
    e False

    The following pharyngeal arches and cranial nerves are paired: arch 1 and trigeminal nerve; arch 2 and facial nerve; arch 3 and glossopharyngeal nerve; arch 4 and vagus nerve; arch 6 and recurrent laryngeal nerve. Arch 1 forms Meckel's cartilage.

---

39. **α-Adrenergic blocking agents**

    a True
    b False
    c False
    d True
    e False

---

40. **The following structures lie posterior to the grey line of the eyelid**

    a True
    b True
    c True
    d False
    e False

    The glands of Zeis and Moll lie anterior to the grey line, as do the lash follicles.

---

41. **The arterial supply to the retina**

    a True
    b False
    c True
    d False
    e False

The retina receives two sources of blood supply, from choroidal capillaries and from the central retinal artery. There are no arteriovenous anastamoses, and no lymph vessels in the retina. The foveal avascular zone is 500 μm in diameter.

42. The roof of the fourth ventricle is formed by

a True
b True
c False
d True
e False

The superior medullary velum is a thin layer of white matter which assists in covering the roof of the fourth ventricle.

43. With regard to ocular neovascularization

a True
b True
c False
d True
e True

Vascular endothelial growth factor (VEGF) is an angiogenic factor provided on retinal capillary endothelial cells and is found in increased quantities in the vitreous and aqueous in ocular ischaemia. Ocular neovascularization occurs as a response to a wide range of insults, including inflammatory eye disease. Corticosteroids are anti-angiogenic.

44. The hyaloid artery

a True
b False
c False
d False
e True

The hyaloid artery develops in concert with the venous system during fetal development, and it develops branches that form the central retinal artery. It regresses in the third trimester and is no longer patent and loses its connection to the optic disk at month 7. It may persist as a remnant at the optic disk and is called Bergmeister's papilla.

45. **Benign tumours that form within epithelial tissue feature**

   a True
   b True
   c True
   d True
   e False

   In a junctional naevus, melanocytic proliferation is confined to the basal layer of the epidermis and a flat patch is seen clinically.

46. **Regarding laboratory tests in HIV infection**

   a True
   b False
   c True
   d True
   e True

   Western blotting demonstrates IgM and IgG against envelope protein and structural protein coded for by the *gag* gene. The earliest laboratory finding is p24 (core protein) anti-genaemia, followed after about 2–3 weeks by an antibody response.

47. **Examples of RNA viruses include**

   a True
   b True
   c True
   d True
   e False

48. **Botulinum toxin type A**

   a False
   b True
   c True
   d False
   e True

Botulinum toxin type A is one of eight serotypes produced by the anaerobic bacterium *Clostridium botulinum*. It non-competitively blocks neurotransmission at the motor end-plate, by blocking the release of acetylcholine.

49. Chronic inflammation

a True
b False
c False
d False
e True

50. *Acanthamoeba*

a False
b True
c True
d True
e True

Acanthamoeba requires selective culture with *E.coli*-seeded agar plates. It is a free-living organism, and may cause granulomatous encephalitis. The amoebae form trophozoites and cysts, which are used for diagnosis in tissue biopsies.

51. *Chlamydia trachomatis*

a True
b False
c False
d False
e True

Chlamydia cannot grow on inanimate media. The bacteria grow well in cell culture (McCoy media). They cannot make ATP and require host metabolites to replicate in host cytoplasm. Inclusion bodies are basophilic.

52. Dense regular connective tissue contains

a True
b True
c False

d True
e True

All connective tissue contains cells, fibres and amorphous ground substance. Dense regular connective tissue contains few cells and many fibres.

---

53. **The transport of molecules across the lens surface**

a True
b True
c True
d False
e False

The Na^+/K^+ ATPase pump is present in the lens epithelium. Chloride ions and water are transferred by passive diffusion.

---

54. **Levator palpebrae superioris**

a True
b False
c False
d True
e False

It originates from the lesser wing of the sphenoid bone and is attached to the medial and lateral palpebral ligaments and also to the tarsal plate. It raises the upper lid by 12–13 mm in adults.

---

55. **In response to infection and inflammation the acquired immune system includes**

a True
b True
c False
d False
e True

The acquired immune system includes mucosal-associated lymphoid tissue (MALT), antibodies, and cytokines, whereas the innate immune system includes physicochemical barriers (skin, tears, eyelids), some molecules within body fluids (e.g.

complement), and phagocytic cells such as polymorphs, eosinophils, and natural killer cells.

56. The central retinal artery

a True
b False
c True
d True
e False

It is the first branch of the ophthalmic artery.

57. Optic nerve glioma

a True
b False
c False
d False
e False

Usually the globe is displaced down and out, and upward movement is markedly limited. The condition is only bilateral in neurofibromatosis. Psammoma bodies are a feature of optic nerve meningioma. Flexner–Wintersteiner rosettes are characteristic of (but not always present in) retinoblastoma.

58. Acute inflammatory processes

a True
b False
c False
d False
e True

Neutrophils predominate initially, but after 24–48 hours are replaced by monocytes. The globe and orbit lack anatomically defined lymphatics. Leucocytes first make contact with the endothelium (margination) and then clump in large numbers (adhesion).

59. The tear film

a False
b True
c True
d False
e True

The tear film is about 10 μm thick. The lipid layer is very thin compared to the aqueous layer.

60. A polymorphonuclear leucocytic infiltrate is a feature of infection by

a False
b False
c False
d True
e True

Paper 2 – Answers

ANSWERS

1. Glutamate

a True
b False
c False
d False
e True

Glutamate activates NMDA receptors, and is excitatory to horizontal cells.

2. The following diseases are inherited in an X-linked fashion

a False
b True
c True
d True
e True

Ocular albinism is inherited in an X-linked fashion, whereas oculocutaneous albinism is autosomal recessive. Other X-linked disorders include red–green colour blindness and blue cone monochromacy.

3. G proteins

a True
b True
c False
d True
e True

G proteins are so called because of their affinity for guanine nucleotides. They play a role in transmitting signals to cell messengers or ion channels, and are thought to play a role in intraocular pressure control.

4. The following are features of mitochondrial diseases

a False
b True
c False
d True
e False

There is no transmission from males to their offspring. In Leber's hereditary optic neuropathy there is an amino acid point mutation in NADH (arginine to histidine). Tissues most reliant on oxygen include the heart, CNS, kidneys, and endocrine organs and these are the most affected by mitochondrial disease.

---

5. **The innervation of the lacrimal apparatus**

   a False
   b True
   c True
   d True
   e False

The pterygopalatine ganglion only provides parasympathetic fibres. The retro-orbital plexus gives out rami lacrimales which carry nonmyelinated postganglionic fibres.

---

6. **The structure of the tear film**

   a False
   b False
   C True
   d True
   e True

An outer lipid layer is present. The aqueous layer is formed mainly by the main lacrimal gland, much less being derived from the named accessory glands of Krause and Wolfring. Blinks disrupt and reform the tear film about 12 to 15 times a minute.

---

7. **Toxic effects of aminoglycoside antibiotics include**

   a True
   b True
   c True
   d True
   e False

---

8. **Retinal ganglion cells**

   a False
   b True

c **True**
d **True**
e **True**

Retinal ganglion cells transmit impulses faster in larger diameter axons. They mediate the transmission of spatially coded signals. Ninety per cent contribute axons that form the parvocellular system. The magnocellular system encodes non-colour information, whereas the parvocellular system encodes high spatial frequency information.

9. **Crystallins within the lens**

a **False**
b **True**
c **True**
d **False**
e **True**

Crystallins constitute 90% of the total protein content of the lens. They are important in maintaining the transparency of the lens. High-molecular-weight aggregates may accumulate with age but this decreases transparency. In a 'typical' lens, the α crystallins predominate.

10. **Genetic and acquired defects in DNA**

a **False**
b **True**
c **False**
d **False**
e **True**

If a purine changes to another purine, or a pyrimidine to another pyrimidine, the point mutation is called a transition. If a purine changes to a pyrimidine or vice versa, the mutation is a transversion. Transitions outnumber transversions at most human loci where naturally occurring mutations have been characterized. A nonsense mutation, also called a premature stop codon, is one that changes a codon that normally specifies an amino acid as a termination codon (this is known to occur in one form of hereditary retinoblastoma). A frameshift mutation occurs when one or more bases are

89

inserted into or deleted from the coding region of a gene. A frameshift mutation changes the reading frame of the encoded message.

---

11. **In Horner's syndrome**

   a True
   b False
   c True
   d True
   e False

---

12. **In Adie's pupil**

   a False
   b False
   c True
   d True
   e False

Features of Holmes–Adie syndrome include a dilated pupil (in the early stages), vermiform pupil movements, a poor response to light and to near, and diminished or absent deep tendon reflexes.

---

13. **Mucosal associated lymphoid tissue**

   a True
   b True
   c True
   d True
   e False

Mucosal associated lymphoid tissue is not limited by capsule.

---

14. **The following HLA types and diseases are associated**

   a False
   b False
   c True
   d True
   e True

---

15. In X-linked dominant inheritance

a False
b True
c True
d False
e False

The risk of a mother having an affected child is 50%. Affected children of an affected father are all female. Christmas disease is X-linked recessive.

---

16. Conjunctival tissue

a True
b True
c True
d True
e True

---

17. Cranial neural crest gives rise to

a False
b False
c True
d True
e True

Extraocular muscle fibres arise from mesoderm. Neuro-sensory retina forms from a thickening of neural ectoderm (known as the retinal disk). Neural crest cells contribute significantly to bone, cartilage, connective tissues, and meninges.

---

18. The Golgi apparatus

a True
b False
c True
d False
e True

Ribosomes are membrane bound on rough endoplasmic reticulum, not the Golgi apparatus. Smooth and rough endoplasmic reticulum both interact with the Golgi apparatus, contributing to the forming face of the Golgi apparatus. mRNA for protein synthesis is bound to rough endoplasmic reticulum.

19. **Complement activation**

a **False**
b **True**
c **False**
d **False**
e **True**

Complement activation is regulated at all stages. Lectins (forming the recently described 'third pathway') activate complement via the classic pathway. An antibody–antigen combination is required to activate the classic pathway.

20. **Media required for incubating micro-organisms include**

a **False**
b **True**
c **True**
d **True**
e **True**

Thioglycolate broth is for both aerobic and anaerobic bacteria, and is used as a general all-purpose medium. *Neisseria* and *Haemophilus* species are fastidious and require an enriched culture medium (chocolate agar).

21. **The flash electroretinogram**

a **False**
b **True**
c **True**
d **False**
e **False**

Ganzfeld stimulation produces uniform illumination to the entire retina. The 'a' wave (generated by photoreceptors) is negative polarity. The 'b' wave is derived from inner retinal elements.

22. Benzalkonium chloride

a True
b False
c True
d False
e True

Benzalkonium chloride is a surfactant preservative which attains it bactericidal activity by attaching to bacterial cell walls, increasing permeability, and causing cell rupture. It is most effective at a slightly alkaline pH, but is inactivated by calcium and magnesium. It may cause papillary conjunctivitis or punctate keratitis.

23. The following enzyme(s) are abundant in the Golgi apparatus

a False
b False
c False
d False
e True

HMG-CoA reductase is an endoplasmic reticular enzyme involved in cholesterol synthesis. Sialyl transferase is a Golgi apparatus enzyme that adds sialic acid residues to glycoproteins.

24. Immunoglobulin subclasses

a True
b True
c True
d False
e True

25. Thiazide diuretics

a False
b True
c True
d False
e True

Thiazide diuretics are actively secreted into the prox-
imal convoluted tubule. They may decrease glomerular fil-
tration (and exacerbate existing renal failure), and they
slightly increase urine pH. They weakly inhibit carbonic
anhydrase, but diuresis is not dependent on this mechanism.

26. Ciliary body epithelium

a **True**
b **True**
c **False**
d **False**
e **False**

Adrenergic α_2 and β_2 receptors predominate. Pilocarpine
increases aqueous outflow by causing ciliary muscle to pull
on the trabecular meshwork.

27. The following are parametric tests

a **True**
b **False**
c **True**
d **False**
e **False**

Parametric data are normally distributed, nonparametric
data are categorical. The Student t-test is used to compare
two normally distributed populations, as is the analysis of
variance test (or ANOVA) which compares more than two
groups. Chi-square and Fisher Exact tests analyse categorical
data (e.g. a two-by-two table).

28. Nonsteroidal anti-inflammatory agents such as aspirin

a **False**
b **True**
c **True**
d **True**
e **False**

Aspirin inhibits prostaglandin synthesis by inhibiting cyclo-
oxygenase. Overdose is treated with acetylcysteine.

29. **In lymph nodes**

    a True
    b True
    c False
    d True
    e True

    Lymph nodes contain B cells in primary and secondary nodules, and T cells in deep tertiary cortex. Secondary nodules allow plasma cell formation from B cells. Reticular fibres exist throughout lymph nodes.

30. **Features of macrophages include**

    a False
    b False
    c True
    d False
    e True

    Each macrophage has numerous microfilaments (for motility). They are phagocytes and have numerous surface projections and lysosomes. The nucleus has an irregular shape.

31. **Interleukin 1**

    a True
    b True
    c True
    d True
    e True

    Interleukin has many roles: lymphocyte activator, endogenous pyrogen, fibroblast stimulator.

32. **The normal corneal endothelium**

    a False
    b False
    c False
    d False
    e False

The normal corneal endothelium comprises approximately 350 000 cells (approximately 3000 cells/mm^2). Cell density declines steadily with age. The endothelium is important in maintaining cornea clarity; however, endothelial cells pump water and ions out of the cornea, reducing its thickness. The initial homogeneous cell population of the endothelium becomes heterogeneous because some cells enlarge with ageing, whereas others do not.

33. The lacrimal gland

a **True**
b **True**
c **False**
d **False**
e **False**

The orbital portion makes up two thirds of the gland. Sympathetic supply is from the deep petrosal nerve, which synapses in the superior cervical ganglion.

34. The tear film

a **True**
b **False**
c **False**
d **True**
e **True**

The tear film pH is a little alkaline at pH 7.5.

35. Delayed type IV hypersensitivity

a **True**
b **False**
c **True**
d **False**
e **False**

36. Tetracyclines

a **True**
b **False**
c **False**

d True
e True

They bind to the 30s subunit and inhibit chain termination.

---

37. Vitamin A

a True
b True
c False
d False
e True

Chylomicrons pass to the liver from the gut. Vitamin A is carried in the bloodstream by prealbumin.

---

38. The following drugs act at the postsynaptic motor endplate

a True
b False
c False
d False
e False

Latrotoxin (Black Widow spider venom) causes excessive release of acetylcholine, whereas botulinum toxin interferes with the release of acetylcholine from the pre-synaptic end plate. Hemicolinium affects choline uptake presynaptically. Atropine blocks muscarinic cholinergic receptors, with little effect on cholinergic transmission at autonomic ganglia and neuromuscular junctions.

---

39. The iris

a True
b True
c True
d True
e False

Full pigmentation is not complete until a few years postpartum. Sphincter fibres develop before dilator fibres (which develop much later at around 6 months).

40. Cerebrospinal fluid

a False
b True
c True
d False
e False

The pH is 7.3 compared with 7.4 for blood. CSF is actively secreted by choroid plexuses.

41. Neutrophil granulocytes

a True
b True
c True
d True
e False

Neutrophils have a life span of less than a day. Glucocorticoids suppress levels of lymphocytes and eosinophils. Granulocytes are formed in the bone marrow.

42. Blockade of parasympathetic activity causes an increase in

a True
b False
c False
d False
e True

Resting heart rate increases due to blockade of vagal tone. Sweat glands are innervated by sympathetic cholinergic nerves. Parasympathetic nerves are not involved in skeletal muscle contraction.

43. The vitreous gel

a True
b True
c False
d False
e True

Vitreous has a refractive index of 1.33 and transmits 90% of visible light. It contains 98% water, 1% hyaluronic acid and type II collagen. Type IX collagen is also a constitutent.

---

44. **Cells of the retinal pigment epithelium**

    a False
    b False
    c True
    d True
    e False

    They form a single layer of hexagonal cells, decline in number with age, and are larger in the periphery.

---

45. **The following peptides are synthesized by neurosecretory neurones originating from the hypothalamus**

    a False
    b True
    c False
    d False
    e False

    Somatostatin is a hypophysiotropic hormone produced from parvicellular neurones; it stimulates the release of growth hormone from the pituitary. Somatomedin is a hepatic hormone.

---

46. **Aqueous humour**

    a False
    b False
    c True
    d False
    e True

    Anterior chamber volume = 0.25 ml. Posterior chamber volume = 0.06 ml. Aqueous is composed predominantly of electrolytes and low-molecular-weight compounds with some protein, but several trace compounds are also present. These compounds include steroid sex hormones, carbonic anhydrase, fibroblast growth factor, and transforming growth factor β. Low levels of catecholamines, prostaglandins, and cyclic nucleotides are present.

---

47. Drugs that may increase intraocular pressure include

a False
b False
c True
d True
e True

---

48. Local anaesthetics

a False
b True
c False
d True
e False

Lidocaine (lignocaine) is also a class I anti-arrhythmic agent (binding to open sodium channels), but has no negative inotropic action. Hypersensitivity reactions are extremely rare, but when they occur are associated mainly with the ester-type local anaesthetics such as tetracaine (amethocaine) and procaine; reactions are less frequent with the amide types such as lidocaine (lignocaine) and bupivacaine.

---

49. When light strikes a photoreceptor outer segment

a False
b False
c True
d False
e True

Rhodopsin is activated. Under resting conditions, sodium leaks into the extracellular space, but when light strikes the photoreceptor, the sodium channels abruptly stop the outflow of sodium, leading to a reduced level of depolarization, i.e. a relative hyperpolarization. cGMP keeps sodium channels open.

---

50. The ciliary body

a False
b True

c False
d True
e True

---

51. Desçemet's membrane

a True
b True
c False
d False
e True

This is a thin, discrete, PAS-positive layer between the posterior stroma and endothelium. It is 8 to 10 μm in thickness. The anterior layer is banded.

---

52. Antihistamine drugs

a True
b False
c True
d False
e True

Antihistamines do not prevent the release of histamine from mast cells; they modify the symptoms of histamine release. Anticholinergic side effects include dry mouth, cough, palpitations, and headache.

---

53. The vitreous cavity

a True
b False
c True
d True
e False

Ascorbic acid is present in relatively high concentrations in the vitreous, and this may relate to its ability to absorb ultraviolet light and act as a free radical scavenger. Hyaluronic acid is the major glycosaminoglycan in the vitreous.

54. Vertical nystagmus

a True
b False
c True
d False
e True

Drug toxicity may cause nystagmus in any direction. If the fast phase is down beating, the lesion is usually low in the medulla, and may be caused by an Arnold–Chiari malformation. There may be oscillopsia present (a sensation of the visual field moving up and down).

55. The following are components of the electroretinogram

a True
b True
c True
d True
e True

The negative 'a' wave is generated by hyperpolarization of photoreceptor inner segments (Granit's PIII component); the 'a' wave is split into a1 and a2 components (cones and rods respectively). The early receptor potential is the first detectable electrical response (which is difficult to record). Oscillatory potentials are thought to be generated by amacrine cells.

56. The polymerase chain reaction

a True
b False
c False
d False
e True

The polymerase chain reaction is a technique that allows small amounts of DNA to be amplified for detection and analysis. Synthetic primers are used to trigger the amplification process.

57. Class II major histocompatibility complex molecules

a False
b True
c True
d True
e True

Class I and class II molecules are membrane bound heterodimers. Class II molecules link to β_2 microglobulin. They both consist of α and β pleated sheets.

58. The following antibiotics inhibit cell wall synthesis

a True
b True
c False
d True
e False

Sulphonamides inhibit folate synthesis. Erythromycin disrupts protein synthesis by binding to ribosomal subunits and interferes with translocation.

59. Advantages of sterilization by autoclave include

a True
b True
c False
d True
e True

60. Cytokine mediators

a False
b False
c True
d False
e True

Cytokines are proteins not lipoproteins. Interleukin-3 is a pan- specific haemopoetin. T cell subsets make different lymphokines, for example T1 helper cells secrete interleukin-2 and interferon-γ whereas T2 helper cells secrete IL-4, -5 and -10.

Paper 3 – Answers

ANSWERS

---

1. **The ciliary ganglion**

   a False
   b True
   c False
   d True
   e True

   It receives three roots. The parasympathetic fibres are the only ones to form synapses.

---

2. **Regarding features of the cornea**

   a True
   b False
   c True
   d True
   e True

   Type I and type III collagen are predominant within corneal stroma. Bowman's layer is not a membrane, and it contains no cells; it is formed from a modified acellular region of stroma.

---

3. **The lacrimal gland**

   a False
   b True
   c False
   d True
   e True

   The lacrimal gland measures approximately 20 mm by 12 mm by 5 mm.

---

4. **The optic tracts**

   a True
   b True
   c True
   d False
   e True

5. *Streptococcus pneumoniae*

a False
b True
c False
d True
e False

The capsule is the only significant virulence factor. *Streptococcus pneumoniae* is α-haemolytic.

6. **The contents of the anterior triangle of the neck include**

a True
b True
c True
d False
e False

The third part of the subclavian artery lies in the posterior triangle.

7. **Neural crest**

a True
b True
c False
d True
e False

The corneal epithelium is derived from surface ectoderm. Neural crest cells migrate from anterior mesencephalic and diencephalic regions along the dorsum of the embryo. Neural crest cells do not arise from the forebrain region.

8. **Concerning the development of the face**

a True
b True
c False
d True
e True

Facial development starts from about week 4 and is largely complete by the 10th week. The nasolacrimal groove on each side lies along the line of fusion of the maxillary process with the natural nasal swelling.

9. Concerning the development of the cornea

a False
b True
c False
d False
e True

The first wave of cells forms the corneal endothelium. The intermediate layer of wing cells does not appear until the 4th or 5th month. The maturation of collagen bundles into highly organized lamellae starts in the posterior cornea.

10. The following are derived from the 2nd pharyngeal arch

a True
b True
c True
d False
e True

The 2nd pharyngeal arch derivatives include the epithelial lining of the tonsils, the stapes and greater hyoid bones, and the stylohyoid ligament. Other derivatives include the facial nerve and muscles of facial expression, the posterior belly of digastric and stapedius. The parathyroid gland is derived from the third and fourth arches.

11. Development of vitreous

a False
b True
c False
d True
e True

Primary vitreous forms at 5 weeks. Secondary vitreous is avascular.

12. **Regarding the development of the optic nerve**

    a True
    b True
    c False
    d True
    e True

    Bergmeister's papilla represents glial cells and hyaloid remnants which may persist in the region of the optic nerve head.

13. **The superior oblique muscle**

    a False
    b False
    c True
    d False
    e True

    It arises from the sphenoid bone superomedial to the optic foramen, and acts on the globe at an angle of 54 degrees to the vertical plane. The IVth nerve supplies the muscle via the upper surface.

14. **Regarding pharyngeal arches**

    a False
    b True
    c True
    d True
    e True

    Arch 3 forms the lower part of the hyoid bone and the inferior parathyroid.

15. **Eosinophil polymorphonuclear leucocytes are present in**

    a False
    b True
    c True
    d True
    e False

16. Deposition of elastic tissue is a feature of

    a False
    b True
    c True
    d True
    e False

17. Pigmentation of tissues follows

    a True
    b True
    c True
    d True
    e False

18. The following cells are known to exhibit reactionary proliferation

    a False
    b True
    c True
    d False
    e True

19. The following systemic diseases can cause intraocular inflammation

    a True
    b True
    c True
    d True
    e True

20. Multinucleate giant cells occur in response to the following infections

    a True
    b True
    c False
    d False
    e False

21. **Metastatic calcification occurs in**

    a False
    b True
    c True
    d True
    e False

22. **Lymphocytic infiltration is a feature of**

    a False
    b True
    c False
    d True
    e True

23. **Tumours derived from epithelial cells can be characterized by**

    a True
    b True
    c False
    d False
    e True

24. **The external carotid artery**

    a False
    b False
    c False
    d False
    e False

    As its origin, the external carotid artery lies medial to the internal carotid artery. Higher up it is situated lateral to this artery. Numerous anastamoses exist between the internal and external carotid circulation. On entering the parotid gland, it lies deep to the facial nerve. The superficial temporal and maxillary arteries are both terminal branches of the external carotid artery.

25. **Melanin pigmentation is observed in**

    a True
    b True
    c True
    d False
    e False

26. **Malignant soft tissue tumours**

    a False
    b True
    c False
    d True
    e False

27. **In temporal arteritis a biopsy may reveal**

    a True
    b True
    c True
    d True
    e True

28. **In which of the following diseases is a necrotizing vasculitis a feature?**

    a False
    b True
    c True
    d True
    e False

29. **The optic chiasma may be compressed by**

    a False
    b True
    c True
    d False
    e False

30. Birefringent crystals are seen in the tissues in

a True
b True
c True
d True
e False

31. Photoreceptor atrophy is a feature of

a False
b True
c True
d True
e False

32. The nerve fibre layer of the retina is atrophic in

a True
b True
c False
d True
e True

33. Corneal development

a False
b True
c True
d False
e True

The first wave of neural crest cells forms endothelium; the second wave forms the iris and pupillary membranes; the third forms keratocytes.

34. Landmarks in retinal development include

a False
b True
c True
d True
e False

Retinal maturation commences at the posterior pole and proceeds towards the periphery.

---

35. Features of the lateral wall of the orbit include

a True
b False
c True
d False
e True

The zygomatic foramen transmits the zygomatic nerve and vessels to the cheek. Spina recti lateralis gives origin to part of the lateral rectus.

---

36. Herpes viruses

a False
b False
c True
d True
e True

Herpes viruses are DNA viruses, and cannot be distinguished by electron microscopy. They may cross the placenta, and cause latent effects including various forms of carcinoma; for example, Epstein–Barr virus is associated with nasopharyngeal carcinoma.

---

37. Actinomycosis infection

a True
b True
c False
d False
e False

Actinomycetes are filamentous Gram-positive bacteria. They have similarities to fungi as they develop hyphae. Spread is via the bloodstream. About two thirds of cases affect the cervicofacial region. Actinomycete infection may cause lacrimal canaliculitis and dacryocystitis, but also severe disseminated infection.

38. β haemolytic streptococci

   a False
   b True
   c True
   d True
   e True

   The Lancefield grouping for streptococci uses different anti-gens on bacterial polysaccharide coats as a means of identi-fication.

39. *Cytomegalovirus* infection

   a True
   b True
   c True
   d True
   e True

40. Recognized features of toxoplasmosis include

   a True
   b True
   c True
   d True
   e True

41. *Chlamydia trachomatis*

   a True
   b True
   c True
   d True
   e False

42. Meningococcal infection

   a False
   b True
   c True
   d False
   e False

Meningococci are Gram-negative diplococci. Reported notifications have increased in recent years but incidence year on year has not risen unduly.

---

43. Concerning the development of the skull

a **True**
b **True**
c **False**
d **True**
e **True**

---

44. Lens development

a **False**
b **True**
c **False**
d **False**
e **True**

Induction occurs at about day 27. Secondary lens fibres arise from the anterior epithelium.

---

45. Sclera

a **False**
b **True**
c **False**
d **True**
e **False**

Sclera contains ill-defined layers (episclera, sclera proper (stroma), lamina fusca), and consists of collagen types I and III predominantly.

---

46. *Staphylococcus aureus*

a **True**
b **True**
c **True**
d **True**
e **True**

47. The anterior lamella of the upper lid

a **False**
b **True**
c **True**
d **False**
e **False**

The eyelid can be split into anterior and posterior lamellae. The anterior lamella (skin, fat, orbicularis) provides little eyelid support; instead the tarsus from the posterior lamella provides the mechanical support. The ciliary glands of Moll lie anterior to the grey line. The eyelashes are modified hairs, with no arrector pili muscle.

48. The ophthalmic artery

a **False**
b **False**
c **False**
d **True**
e **False**

The ophthalmic artery is a branch of the internal carotid artery. It arises after the internal carotid artery has passed through the cavernous sinus and lies below and lateral to the optic nerve in the optic canal. The ophthalmic artery arises in the middle cranial fossa, and lies medial to the anterior clinoid process.

49. *Staphylococcus aureus*

a **False**
b **True**
c **False**
d **True**
e **True**

50. DNA viruses

a **False**
b **False**
c **False**
d **False**
e **False**

DNA viruses usually contain linear double-stranded DNA. Adenovirus is a DNA virus, but hepatitis A is an RNA virus.

---

51. Features of the floor of the middle cranial fossa include

a **False**
b **True**
c **False**
d **True**
e **False**

The optic canal lies between the two roots of the lesser wing of the sphenoid. The foramen rotundum transmits the maxillary nerve and small veins from the cavernous sinus. The foramen spinosum is posterolateral to foramen ovale, and transmits the middle meningeal artery and vein, and the meningeal branch of the mandibular nerve.

---

52. The following pass through the foramen magnum

a **False**
b **False**
c **True**
d **True**
e **True**

The vertebral arteries pass through the foramen magnum (to form the basilar artery superiorly).

---

53. Gonococcal infection

a **True**
b **True**
c **False**
d **False**
e **True**

About 1 in 700 cases have ophthalmic involvement. Transmission is from the genitalia to the hand to the eye. Conjunctival pseudomembranes may form.

54. The choroid

a **True**
b **True**
c **False**
d **False**
e **True**

Pigment-bearing melanocytes appear at around month 7–8.

55. In the 10-week-old embryo

a **False**
b **False**
c **False**
d **False**
e **False**

The approximate length is 50 mm. Myelination of the optic nerve begins at around 7 months. Ciliary muscle develops at about 4 months. Retinal differentiation begins at 6 weeks.

56. Mesoderm derivatives include

a **True**
b **True**
c **True**
d **True**
e **True**

57. The following are derived from the 2nd pharyngeal arch

a **False**
b **False**
c **True**
d **False**
e **False**

Thyroid cartilage forms from the 4th arch. Incus and malleus form from the 1st arch, stylopharyngeus from the 3rd.

58. Corneal stroma

a False
b True
c False
d False
e True

Corneal stroma contains predominantly type I collagen.

59. Onchocerciasis

a True
b True
c False
d True
e True

Microfilaria migrate subcutaneously through the body. Molecular mimicry occurs as host T cells recognize cross-reactive antigens on *Onchorcerca* and retinal proteins.

60. Lipopolysaccharide

a True
b True
c True
d True
e True

Endotoxins are lipopolysaccharides derived from the cell wall composed of lysed or dead Gram-negative bacteria upon autolysis. Unlike exotoxins they are heat stable. Lipopolysaccharide may cause fever and induce complement.

Paper 4 – Answers

ANSWERS

---

1. **Restriction endonuclease enzymes**

   a **True**
   b **True**
   c **True**
   d **True**
   e **True**

   Restriction endonucleases cut DNA at specific recognition sites, and may be used to identify polymorphisms. In Southern blotting, a DNA sample is cut into several fragments by restriction endonucleases, and denatured into single strands. Pre-prepared radiolabelled DNA probes are used to determine any matches with the single-stranded DNA, by identification with autoradiography.

---

2. **Characteristic features of Turner syndrome include**

   a **False**
   b **True**
   c **True**
   d **True**
   e **True**

   The karyotype is XO. Other cardiac features include aortic coarctation, bicuspid aortic valve. Affected individuals are usually short. Cubitus valgus produces the 'wide carrying angle'.

---

3. **Autosomal dominant conditions include**

   a **True**
   b **True**
   c **True**
   d **False**
   e **False**

   Macular corneal dystrophy and familial ectopia lentis are recessively inherited.

4. **The following diseases are autosomal recessive**

   a   False
   b   True
   c   True
   d   True
   e   True

   Meesman's corneal dystrophy is autosomal dominant.

5. **Mitochondrial DNA**

   a   False
   b   False
   c   True
   d   False
   e   True

   Mitochondrial DNA is circular. The genetic code for the translation mechanism differs from the 'universal' code. Genetic transmission is thought to be predominantly maternal. Mitochondrial DNA is present in sperm in small quantities but is degraded at conception, and as a result almost all mitochondrial DNA in humans is derived from maternal DNA.

6. **The cornea is transparent because**

   a   False
   b   False
   c   True
   d   False
   e   False

   Collagen fibres within the cornea are predominantly of type I, with some type III, V, and VI. Bowman's layer consists of fine, randomly arranged collagen fibrils.

7. **Concerning the mechanisms of colour vision**

   a   True
   b   False
   c   False
   d   True
   e   True

The opponent theory is based on the receptive field organization of ganglion cells and accommodates the Young–Helmholtz trichromatic theory. The magnocellular pathway deals with light and motion detection (M ganglion cells with large receptive fields) whereas the parvocellular pathway deals with spatial and colour vision (P cells with small receptive fields). The prestriate region V4 contains cells that act as wavelength discriminators.

---

8. **Regarding electrolytes in the cornea**

   a **True**
   b **True**
   c **False**
   d **True**
   e **True**

   The epithelial potassium concentration is approximately 140 mmol/l. Relative to plasma, epithelial concentrations of sodium are lower, potassium higher, and chloride lower. In contrast, when compared to plasma, stromal sodium concentrations are relatively high.

---

9. **Recognized features of trisomy 13 (Patau syndrome)**

   a **True**
   b **True**
   c **True**
   d **True**
   e **True**

   Trisomy 13 (Patau syndrome) illustrates various forms of malformation. The cornea and anterior chamber angle are malformed and persistent hyperplastic primary vitreous is common. An anterior coloboma is present. Retinal dysplasia is extensive, and the optic nerve is hypoplastic. The systemic malformations are not compatible with survival.

---

10. **The antibiotic vancomycin**

    a **False**
    b **False**
    c **True**
    d **False**
    e **True**

Vancomycin is primarily effective against Gram-positive cocci. It is not used routinely in ocular irrigation fluids because of the emerging threat of vancomycin resistance. It works by inhibiting cell wall synthesis, and is excreted by the kidneys.

11. Bruch's membrane

a True
b True
c True
d False
e False

Bruch's membrane separates the basal surface of the retinal pigment epithelium from its blood supply, the choriocapillaris. Bruch's membrane contains open spaces and the basement membrane of the choriocapillaris has discontinuities; therefore Bruch's membrane does not obstruct the passage of macromolecules. With advancing age, the retinal pigment epithelium by-products accumulate and its thickness increases with age.

12. Müller cells

a True
b True
c True
d True
e False

Müller cells are the principal supporting glial cells of the retina. They help to nourish and maintain the outer retina, which lacks a direct blood supply. Müller cells are believed to contribute to 'b' not 'a' waves of the electroretinogram. 'a' Waves are generated by the hyperpolarization of photoreceptor inner segments.

13. Over 120 million rods and 6 millions cones form the neurosensory retina. Which of the following statements is/are correct?

a False
b True

c **True**
d **False**
e **False**

Rod density does in general increase with increasing distance from the fovea (rods are absent at the fovea) but diminish in numbers at the far periphery. Rod density is greatest immediately temporal to the optic disk ($170\,000/mm^2$).

---

14. Mydriatic agents with cycloplegic action include

a **True**
b **True**
c **False**
d **True**
e **False**

Cyclopentolate and homatropine usually cause mydriasis within 30 minutes and cycloplegia within 1 hour. Phenylephrine dilates the pupil without cycloplegia. Physostigmine is a rarely used miotic agent.

---

15. The vital capacity of the lungs

a **True**
b **True**
c **False**
d **False**
e **False**

The vital capacity equals the expiratory reserve volume plus the inspiratory capacity. The inspiratory capacity is the sum of the inspiratory reserve volume and the tidal volume. The residual volume accounts for the difference between the total lung capacity and the vital capacity, normally being about 1.2 litres.

---

16. The null hypothesis

a **True**
b **False**
c **True**
d **False**
e **True**

The null hypothesis is accepted when the alternative hypothesis is true in type II error.

17. **Mitochondria perform the following function(s)**

a **True**
b **True**
c **False**
d **True**
e **True**

Mitochondria synthesize DNA when they replicate and contain enzymes that assist in steroid synthesis. Their main function is to produce ATP via oxidative phosporylation. Enzymes that degrade polysaccharides are found in lysosomes.

18. **The intracellular matrix**

a **False**
b **True**
c **True**
d **True**
e **True**

Microfilaments include actin, troponin, and tropomyosin. They are universal cell constituents and are involved in cell motility and structural integrity. Intermediate filaments are coiled α helices and act as stretchable components of the cytoskeleton scaffold. Vimentin (found in mesenchymal cells) and desmin (found in muscle cells) are intermediate filaments.

19. **Retinal pigment epithelial cells**

a **True**
b **False**
c **False**
d **True**
e **True**

20. **The visual evoked potential**

a **True**
b **False**

c True
d False
e True

The visual evoked potential measures the gross electrical response of the cerebral cortex to visual stimulation. Scalp electrodes are positioned over the primary occipital visual area.

---

21. Antigen presentation

    a True
    b True
    c True
    d False
    e True

T cells only recognize processed antigen in association with MHC molecules.

---

22. Endotoxins

    a True
    b False
    c False
    d True
    e True

---

23. Human housekeeping genes

    a True
    b False
    c False
    d True
    e True

The basal metabolic activity of a cell depends on the transcription of housekeeping genes. In comparison to genes that are expressed primarily in a specific tissue or during a particular phase of development, the expression level of a housekeeping gene remains relatively constant.

24. Stimulation of renin secretion

a False
b True
c False
d False
e False

Renin is an enzyme that catalyses the reaction that forms angiotensin I from angiotensinogen. Angiotensin I, in turn, is converted to angiotensin II by angiotensin converting enzyme. Angiotensin II is a potent vasoconstrictor and stimulates release of aldosterone from the adrenals, causing increased extracellular fluid volume through increased sodium reabsorption in the kidney.

25. Non-parametric statistical tests are used to

a False
b False
c False
d True
e False

The unpaired t test and regression calculations which require continuous data involve parametric tests. The Fisher Exact test is used instead of the chi-square test for small sample sizes.

26. Glycogen synthesis

a True
b True
c True
d True
e True

In the liver, glycogen may be formed from glucose (requiring glucokinase) or lactate.

27. Glucose transport by insulin-dependent facilitated diffusion occurs in

a True
b True

c **True**

d **False**

e **False**

---

28. **Collagen type I**

a **True**

b **False**

c **False**

d **False**

e **False**

Type I collagen is found in bone, tendon, skin, and cornea. It consists of two α_1 chains and one α_2 chain. Type II collagen is most abundant in cartilage and vitreous. Type IV collagen is most abundant in basement membranes. Type V collagen is found in basement membranes that surround smooth-muscle cells.

---

29. **Varicella zoster virus**

a **False**

b **False**

c **True**

d **True**

e **False**

The following viruses are associated with cancer: (1) Epstein–Barr virus with Burkitt's lymphoma and nasopharyngeal carcinoma; (2) human papilloma virus with cervical carcinoma; (3) hepatitis B virus with liver carcinoma; (4) HIV with Kaposi's sarcoma and non-Hodgkin's lymphoma. VZV is a double-stranded DNA virus.

---

30. **The pattern electroretinogram**

a **False**

b **False**

c **False**

d **True**

e **True**

Pattern reversal occurs at 1–2 Hz. Signal amplitude is about 2–4 mV. The signal is generated in the retina.

31. The neurohypophysis contains the following cell types

a False
b False
c False
d False
e False

The pituitary gland consists of the adenohypophysis and neurohypophysis. The former contains basophils, acidophils, and chromophobes. Gonadotrophs are one kind of basophil; lactotrophs are one kind of acidophil. Chromophobes are found within the adenohypophysis and stain poorly. The neurohypophysis contains pituicytes, which are glial cells interspersed between the nerve processes originating in the median eminence.

32. In Horner's syndrome

a True
b True
c True
d True
e False

Horner's syndrome consists of mild ptosis, miosis, and a variable degree of sweating on the affected side. The sympathetic outflow to the pupils is at level T_1, and therefore Horner's syndrome may be caused by lower trunk brachial plexus lesions. Hydroxyamphetamine drops release noradrenaline (norepinephrine) from functional terminal axons and therefore dilate the pupil if the lesion is central or preganglionic, but not postganglionic (because the axon is not functional).

33. In type II hypersensitivity

a False
b True
c True
d True
e True

34. Autosomal dominant conditions

a False
b True
c True
d False
e True

35. Rhodopsin

a True
b False
c True
d True
e False

Rhodopsin is an integral membrane protein.

36. Angle-closure glaucoma may be in part precipitated by

a False
b True
c False
d True
e True

Antimuscarinic agents may cause dilatation of the pupil, and precipitate acute glaucoma.

37. T lymphocytes produce the following cytokines

a False
b True
c True
d True
e True

T lymphocytes secrete interleukin-2 and -3 (and other interleukins), but interleukin-1 is secreted by macrophages. T lymphocytes also activate macrophages by producing macrophage-activating factors such as TNF-α.

38. **Complement activation is regulated by**

    a True
    b True
    c True
    d False
    e False

    Red cell lysis is one possible end result of complement activation.

39. **With respect to epithelial cell turnover**

    a True
    b True
    c False
    d True
    e True

40. **Class I major histocompatibility complex molecules**

    a True
    b False
    c True
    d True
    e True

41. **In X-linked recessive conditions**

    a False
    b True
    c False
    d False
    e True

42. **The corneal stroma**

    a False
    b False
    c True
    d False
    e True

The corneal stroma contains about 200 lamellae; each is about 2 μm thick. No anatomically defined lymph vessels are present to help maintain corneal clarity.

---

43. The otic ganglion

a False
b True
c True
d True
e False

The otic ganglion is placed below foramen ovale, and lies below the origin of the maxillary branch of the fifth cranial nerve.

---

44. Intraocular pressure (IOP)

a False
b False
c True
d True
e False

IOP tends to be overestimated by the non-contact tonometer in higher ranges.

---

45. Acetazolamide

a True
b False
c False
d True
e False

Acetazolamide decreases aqueous production by blocking carbonic anhydrase in the ciliary body. It may cause a relative hypokalaemia and hyponatraemia, and hyperchloraemic metabolic acidosis. Other side effects include renal stones (hypercalciuria), drowsiness, and paraesthesia.

46. Human insulin

a False
b True
c False
d True
e False

Human insulin has a plasma half life of less than 9 minutes, is longer acting if less soluble and is formed from two polypeptide chains. A separate C peptide may connect the two insulin chains.

47. Warfarin

a True
b True
c False
d True
e False

Warfarin starts to produce an anticoagulant effect within 8–12 hours. Warfarin metabolism is inhibited by chloramphenicol.

48. β-adrenoceptor blocking drugs

a True
b True
c False
d True
e True

Even selective β blockers slow the heart rate.

49. Mast cells

a True
b False
c True
d True
e False

Mast cells exist in two forms (mucosal and connective tissue mast cells). They differ in their proliferative response to interleukin-3 and granular proteases. Phosphatidylinositol is broken down to form inositol triphosphate after IgE cross-linking, which leads to diacylglycerol production, and an increase in intracellular calcium. Leukotrienes are synthesized afresh and are not preformed.

50. Local anaesthetics

a False
b True
c True
d False
e True

Local anaesthetics inhibit sodium channels and block the initiation and propagation of action potentials. Bupivacaine has a relatively slow onset of action, taking up to 30 minutes for full effect.

51. Glucocorticoids

a False
b True
c False
d True
e False

Glucocorticoids inhibit phospholipase A_2 – the enzyme that releases arachidonic acid. Glucocorticoids stimulate gluconeogenesis, and have immunosuppressive properties, reducing lymphocyte and eosinophil counts.

52. Sulphonamides

a True
b False
c True
d True
e True

Sulphonamides inhibit the metabolism of *p*-aminobenzoic acid to folate. Folate is essential for bacterial metabolism and DNA synthesis.

---

53. The following substances are present in aqueous humour at higher concentrations than in plasma

a False
b True
c True
d False
e False

---

54. Platelet-derived growth factor

a True
b True
c False
d True
e True

There are three forms of platelet-derived growth factor. All exist as dimers of A or B chains.

---

55. Intraocular pressure typically increases with the following

a True
b True
c True
d True
e True

Intraocular pressure increases with age worldwide, except in Japan where intraocular pressure falls with increasing age.

---

56. Confidence intervals

a False
b True
c True
d True
e True

They typically indicate the level of confidence at the 0.95 probability level.

---

57. Red blood cell inclusions

a False
b False
c True
d True
e True

Post-splenectomy, red blood cell inclusions form from DNA/nuclear fragments and are called Howell–Jolly bodies. In glucose-6-phosphate deficiency, denatured haemoglobin deposits are called Heinz bodies.

---

58. Inhibitors of nucleic acid synthesis

a True
b True
c False
d True
e True

Most, for example aciclovir and ganciclovir, are poorly absorbed orally. Amantadine inhibits growth of influenza A viruses by acting as an ion-channel blocker.

---

59. Chloramphenicol

a True
b False
c True
d False
e True

Chloramphenicol works by inhibiting peptidyl transferase, and is excreted by the kidneys. It is particularly useful in rickettsial and anaerobic infections. Chloramphenicol is effective in meningococcal meningitis, and may be used in penicillin allergic patients in this circumstance. The 'grey baby syndrome' occurs in neonates after exposure to excessive doses of chloramphenicol.

60. Fluoroquinolone antibiotics

a True
b False
c False
d False
e True

Quinolones inhibit DNA gyrase. Gram-positive and anaerobic organisms are less susceptible to quinolones. Oral quinolones can cause irreversible damage to developing cartilage and are not recommended for those under 18 years of age.

BIBLIOGRAPHY

This book is a companion revision aid to the textbook *The Eye: Basic Sciences in Practice*, 2e. We have added other important texts to use as a reference to cover the wide and varied aspects of basic science of the eye and visual science.

Albert DM and Jacobiec FA (1999) *Principles and Practice of Ophthalmology. Basic Sciences.* Philadelphia: W.B. Saunders.

Bron AJ, Tripathi R, Warwick R and Marshall J (1997) *Wolff's Anatomy of the Eye and Orbit.* London: Arnold.

Forrester J, Dick A, McMenamin P and Lee W (2001) *The Eye: Basic Sciences in Practice* 2e. Edinburgh: W.B. Saunders.

Ganong WF (1999) *Review of Medical Physiology*, 19th edn. New York: Appleton and Lange

Hart WH (1992) *Adler's Physiology of the Eye*, 9th edn. London: Mosby.

Roitt IM (1997) *Essential Immunology*, 9th edn. Oxford: Blackwell Science.

Sadler TW (2000) *Langman's Medical Embryology*, 8th edn. Philadelphia: Lippincott, Williams and Wilkins.

Snell RS and Lemp MA (1998) *Clinical Anatomy of the Eye* 2nd edn. Boston: Blackwell Science.

Whikehart DR (1994) *Biochemistry of the Eye.* Oxford: Butterworth Heinemann.

Williams PL and Warwick R (1995) *Gray's Anatomy*, 38th edn. Edinburgh: Churchill Livingstone.

Yanoff M and Fine BS (1995) *Ocular Pathology*, 4th edn. London: Mosby–Wolfe.

INDEX

The numbers given refer to page numbers.

Acanthamoeba, 13, 80
accessory glands of Krause and Wolfring, 88
acebutolol, 61, 138
acetazolamide, 60, 137
acetylcholine, 28, 71, 80, 97
  release, 5
acetylcysteine, 94
aciclovir, 63, 141
actin, 54, 130
actinomycosis infection, 42, 115
adenohypophysis, 134
adenosine triphosphate (ATP) production, 54, 130
adenovirus, 45, 118
Adie's pupil, 21, 90
adrenaline, 61, 139
α-adrenergic blocking agents, 10, 77
adrenergic receptors, 24, 94
β-adrenoceptors, 61, 138
AIDS, 43, 116
albinism, ocular/oculocutaneous, 19, 87
aldosterone, 132
allograft rejection, 9, 75
amantadine, 63, 141
amino acid synthesis, 62, 139
p-aminobenzoic acid, 139
aminoglycosides, 20, 88
amyloid, 10
angiotensin, 132
angiotensin converting enzyme (ACE), 132
angiotensinogen, 56, 132
aniridia, 73
annulus of Zinn, 8, 74
antibiotics
  aminoglycoside, 20, 88
  cell wall synthesis inhibition, 31, 103
  fluoroquinolone, 63, 141
  resistance, 3, 53, 128
  vancomycin, 127–8
antibodies, 81
anticoagulation, 138

antigen presentation, 55, 131
antihistamines, 30, 101
antimuscarinic agents, 58, 135
aqueous humour, 29, 62, 99, 139–40
  development, 70
Arnold–Chiari malformation, 30, 101–2
arytenoid cartilage, 6
ascorbate, 62, 139
ascorbic acid, 30, 101
aspirin, 25, 94
ATPase, 52, 127
atropine, 54, 58, 97, 129, 135
autoclave sterilization, 31, 103
autosomal conditions
  dominant, 51, 58, 125, 126, 134
  recessive, 51, 135

β blockers, 138
B cells, 25, 95
bacterial endocarditis, 39, 111
  see also infective endocarditis
basement membranes, 133
basilar artery, 45, 119
basilar sinuses, 5, 69–70
Behçet's disease, 39, 111
benzalkonium chloride, 24, 93
Bergmeister's papilla, 37, 79, 110
Best's disease, 51, 125
black fly, 4, 47, 68, 120
blinks, 88
bone fracture, 9, 76
botulinum toxin, 13, 27, 71, 97
  type A, 71, 79–80
Bowman's layer, 3, 4, 68, 71, 107
  collagen fibrils, 52, 126
  limbus, 5
brachial plexus, 57, 134
Bruch's membrane, 6, 53, 71–2, 128
bupivacaine, 61, 100, 139

calcification
  dystrophic, 9, 75, 76
  metastases, 39, 112
calcium, intracellular, 138

carbonic anhydrase, 52, 99, 137
catecholamines, 99
cavernous sinus, 3, 4, 68–9, 70, 119
CD4+ T cells, 9, 75
CD8+ T cells, 9, 75
cell-mediated cytotoxicity, 57, 134
cell proliferation, reactionary, 38, 111
central retinal artery, 12, 15, 78, 82
  occlusion, 41, 114
cerebrospinal fluid (CSF), 27, 98
cGMP, 100
chi-square test, 25, 94, 132
Chlamydia trachomatis, 13, 43, 80, 116
  sulphonamides, 62, 139
chloramphenicol, 60, 63, 138, 141
chloride ions, 81
  corneal, 52, 127
chocolate agar, 3, 23, 45, 92
choloramphenicol, 141
choriocapillaris, 46, 53, 119, 128
chorioretinitis, congenital, 43, 116
choroid, 46, 119
  mesoderm derivative, 46, 120
choroid plexus, 98
choroidal capillaries, 78
choroidal vessel sclerosis, 41, 114
Christmas disease, 22, 91
chromophobes, 134
chromosome 11, 73
chromosome 17, 7
chylomicrons, 97
ciliary body, 5, 29, 100–1
  carbonic anhydrase blocking, 137
  development, 5, 70
  epithelium, 24, 94
ciliary ganglion, 35, 107
ciliary glands of Moll, 44, 117
ciliary muscle, 5, 94
  development, 46, 120
Clostridium botulinum, 5, 71, 80
clotting factors, 60
collagen, 30, 46, 68, 120
  bundle maturation, 109
  fibres, 4

fibrils in Bowman's layer, 52, 126
  scleral, 59, 136
  type I, 56, 107, 117, 120, 126, 133
  type II, 4, 5, 28, 44, 70, 73, 99, 133
  type III, 107, 117, 126
  type IV, 126, 133
  type V, 133
  type VI, 126
  type IX, 99
coloboma, anterior, 52, 127
colour blindness, complete, 58, 135
colour vision, 52, 126–7
common tendinous ring, 3, 67
complement, 82, 121
  type II hypersensitivity, 57, 134
complement activation, 23, 47, 55, 92, 121, 131
  regulation, 58, 135–6
cones, 53, 128–9
confidence intervals, 62, 140
congenital malformations, trisomy 13, 52, 127
conjunctiva
  pseudomembranes, 45, 119
  tissue, 22, 91
conjunctivitis, benzalkonium chloride, 93
connective tissue, dense regular, 14, 80–1
cornea, 4, 5, 35, 68, 107
  clarity, 96, 136
  development, 36, 41, 109, 114
  electrolytes, 52, 127
  malformation, 52, 127
  stroma, 46, 59, 120, 136
  transparency, 52, 126
  trisomy 13, 127
corneal dystrophy
  macular, 51, 125
  Meesman's, 51, 126
corneal endothelial cells, 4, 69, 96, 109
  interdigitations, 69
corneal endothelium, 95–6

corneal epithelium, 3, 26, 67
  cell turnover, 136
  regeneration, 59, 136
  surface ectoderm, 108
corneal stroma, 120
cranial neural crest, 22, 91
crystal formation, birefringent, 41, 113
crystallins, 7, 21, 72, 89
cubitus valgus, 51, 125
cyclo-oxygenase inhibitors, 94
cyclopentolate, 54, 129
cycloplegia, 129
cysts, amoebic, 80
cytokines, 31, 58, 81, 103–4, 135
Cytomegalovirus infection, 43, 63, 116, 141
cytoplasmic inclusions, 43, 116

dacryocystitis, 115
deer fly, 4, 68
deletions, 21
Desçemet's membrane, 4, 30, 69, 71, 101
  limbus, 5
  mesoderm derivative, 46, 120
desmin, 54, 130
diabetes, 61, 138
diabetic microangiopathy, 8, 74
diabetic retinopathy, 11, 41, 114
diacylglycerol, 138
dilator muscle development, 73
diuretics, thiazide, 24, 93–4
DNA defects, 21, 89–90
DNA gyrase inhibition, 141
DNA polymorphisms, 51, 125
DNA probes, 125
DNA synthesis, 130, 139
DNA viruses, 45, 115, 118

ectopia lentis, familial, 51, 125
elastic tissue deposition, 38, 110–11
electroretinogram, 31, 55, 102, 130
  flash, 23, 92
    Müller cells, 53, 128
    pattern, 57, 133

embolic disease, pulmonary arterioles, 9, 75
embryo
  6-week-old, 6, 72
  10-week-old, 46, 119–20
encephalitis, granulomatous, 80
endoplasmic reticulum, enzymes, 93
endothelium formation, 114
endotoxins, 55, 121, 131
Enterobius vermicularis, 4
enterotoxins, 3
eosinophils, 9, 38, 82, 98, 110
epithelial cell tumours, 112
epithelial cell turnover, 59, 136
epithelial tissue, benign tumours, 79
Epstein–Barr virus (EBV), 115
error, type II, 130
erythromycin, 103
external carotid artery, 40, 112
extracellular matrix, 9, 76
extraocular muscles, 46, 120
  fibres, 91
eyelash follicles, 77
eyelashes, 117
eyelid
  anterior lamella of upper, 44, 117
  grey line, 11, 77, 117

facial development, 36, 108–9
facial nerve, pharyngeal arch, 77
fetal development
  choroid, 46, 119
  ciliary body, 5, 70
  ciliary muscle, 46, 120
  cornea, 36, 41, 109, 114
  face, 36, 108–9
  hyaloid artery, 78
  lens, 44, 117
  optic nerve, 37, 110
  retina, 42, 114, 120
  skull, 43, 116
  vitreous, 37, 109
fetal fissure, 6, 72
fibroblast growth factor, 99

Fisher Exact test, 25, 94, 132
flash electroretinogram, 23
Flexner–Wintersteiner rosettes, 15, 82
fluoroquinolones, 63, 141
folate synthesis inhibition, 103, 139
foramen magnum, 45, 119
foramen ovale, 119, 137
foramen rotundum, 45, 118
foramen spinosum, 45, 119
fourth ventricle roof, 11, 78
foveal avascular zone, 78
frameshift mutation, 21, 89–90
frontal nerve, 74

G proteins, 19, 87
gag gene, 79
ganciclovir, 63, 141
ganglion cells, receptive field organization, 127
Ganzfield stimulation, 23, 92
gene mapping, 51, 125
genetic transmission, 126
giant cells, 13, 42
  multinucleate, 39, 111
glands of Moll and Zeis, 77
glaucoma, 41, 114
  angle-closure, 58, 135
glossopharyngeal nerve, pharyngeal arch, 77
glucocorticoids, 61, 98, 139
glucokinase, 56, 132
glucose, 56, 132
  transport, 132–3
glucose-6-phosphate, 24
  deficiency, 141
glutamate, 19, 87
glycocalyx proteins, 67
glycogen synthesis, 56, 132
glycosaminoglycans, 4, 68, 70
  Graves' disease, 76
  sclera, 5
  vitreous, 7, 30, 101
Golgi apparatus, 23, 91–2
  enzymes, 24, 93
gonadotrophs, 134

gonococcal infection, 45, 119
granulocytes, 98
Graves' disease, 76
grey baby syndrome, 63, 141
growth hormone, 28, 99
guanine nucleotides, 87

haemochromatosis, 76
haemogoblin, denatured, 141
Haemophilus, 92
heart rate, resting, 98
Heinz bodies, 63, 141
hemicolinium, 27, 97
hemidesmosomes, 59, 136
hepatitis A, 45, 118
herpes viruses, 15, 42, 115
hexosaminidase A deficiency, 51, 126
histamine release, 101
HIV infection, laboratory tests, 12, 79
HLA types, 22, 90–1
HMG-CoA reductase, 24, 93
Holmes–Adie syndrome, 90
homatropine, 54, 129
horizontal cells, 87
Horner's syndrome, 21, 57, 90, 134
housekeeping genes, 55, 131
Howell–Jolly bodies, 63, 141
Hox gene expression, 5, 70
human insulin, 137–8
hyaloid artery, 12, 78–9
hyaloid remnants, 110
hyaluronic acid, 4, 68, 73
  vitreous gel, 99, 101
hydroxyamphetamine, 57, 134
hyoid bone, 6, 37, 72, 109, 110
hypersensitivity
  delayed type IV, 26, 96
  local anaesthetic reactions, 100
  type II, 57, 134
hypokalaemia, 137
hyponatraemia, 137
hypothalamus, neurosecretory neurones, 28, 99

Imbert–Fick principle, 60, 137
immune system, acquired, 14, 81–2
immunoglobulin E, 61, 138
immunoglobulin subclasses, 15, 24,
  93
immunosuppression
  glucocorticoids, 139
  graft rejection, 75
inclusion bodies, 57, 80, 133
incubation media, 23, 92
  chocolate agar, 3, 23, 45, 92
incus, 120
infection, 14
  anaerobic, 141
  multinucleate giant cells, 111
infective endocarditis, 3, 36, 68
  subacute, 39, 111
inflammation, 11, 14
  chronic, 13, 80
  intraocular, 39, 111
inflammatory eye disease, 78
inflammatory processes, acute, 15,
  82
influenza A virus, 141
inheritance
  autosomal dominant, 51, 58, 125,
    126, 134
  autosomal recessive, 51, 126
  dominant, 22, 91
  recessive, 59, 125, 136
  X-linked diseases, 19, 22, 59, 87,
    91, 136
insulin, 56, 132
  human, 60, 137–8
insulin-dependent facilitated
    diffusion, 132–3
interleukin 1 (IL-1), 25, 55, 95,
    130, 131
interleukin 2 (IL-2), 58, 135
interleukin 3 (IL-3), 58, 103–4, 135
interleukin 4 (IL-4), 58
interleukins, 103–4
intermediate filaments, 130
internal carotid artery, 3, 4, 67, 69
  anastomoses to external carotid
    artery, 112

branches, 8, 74–5
  ophthalmic artery, 118
intracellular matrix, 54, 130
intraocular pressure, 19, 24, 29, 60,
  87, 137
  age, 140
  drugs increasing, 100
  increase, 62, 140
  overestimation, 60, 137
iris, 7, 27, 73, 97
  development, 70
  formation, 41, 114
  pigmentation, 97
  sphincter fibres, 27, 97
iron deposition, 76
irradiation therapy, 10, 76–7
ischaemia, 10, 76

keratitis, punctate, 93
keratocytes, 41, 46, 114, 120
ketamine, 62, 140

lacrimal apparatus innervation, 20,
  88
lacrimal canaliculitis, 115
lacrimal gland, 26, 35, 88, 96, 107
lacrimal nerve, 74
lactate, 62, 132, 139
lactotrophs, 134
lamina cribrosa, 37, 72
laryngeal cartilages, 72
lateral geniculate bodies, 6, 71
latrotoxin, 27, 97
Leber's hereditary optic
    neuropathy, 19, 88
lectins, 92
lens
  crystallins, 7, 21, 72, 89
  development, 44, 70, 117
  epithelium, 81
  molecule transport, 14, 81
lens fibres, 6, 72
  secondary, 44, 117
leucocytes, 82, 83
  adhesion, 15
leukotrienes, 138

levator palpebrae superioris, 14, 81
lidocaine (lignocaine), 29, 100
limbus, 5, 70–1
lipid A, 47, 55, 121, 131
lipofuscin, 54, 130
lipopolysaccharide, 47, 55, 121, 131
liver, glycogen synthesis, 132
local anaesthetics, 29, 61, 100, 139
loiasis, 68
lung vital capacity, 54, 129
lymph nodes, 25, 95
lymph nodules, secondary, 95
lymphocytes, 61, 98, 139
  see also B cells; T cells
lymphocytic infiltration, 39, 112
lymphokines, 103–4
lysosomes, 55, 130

macrophages, 10, 25, 95
magnocellular system, 20, 52, 89,
  127
major histocompatibility complex
  (MHC) molecules, 131
  class I, 59, 136
  class II, 31, 55, 103, 131
malignancy
  calcium deposition, 76
  herpes viruses, 42, 115
  soft tissue tumours, 40, 112–13
malleus, 6, 10, 120
mandibular nerve, meningeal
  branch, 119
Marfan's syndrome, 58, 135
mast cells, 9, 61, 138
maxillary artery, 112
maxillary nerve, 4, 69, 119
  inferior, 60
McCoy medium, 43, 80
Meckel's cartilage, 10, 77
Meesman's corneal dystrophy, 51,
  126
Meibomian glands, 8, 74
melanin, 3, 67, 73
  pigmentation, 40, 112
melanocytes, 7
  pigment-bearing, 46, 119

proliferation, 79
melanosomes, 55, 130
meningococcal infection, 43, 116
meningococcal meningitis, 141
mesoderm, derivatives, 46, 120
metabolic acidosis,
  hyperchloraemic, 60, 137
metastases, 8, 10, 75, 76
  calcification, 39, 112
microfilaments, 130
β_2-microglobulin, 103
midbrain, 7, 73–4
middle cranial fossa, 45, 118–19
middle meningeal vessels, 60, 119,
  137
mitochondria, 54, 130
mitochondrial diseases, 19, 87–8
mitochondrial DNA, 51, 126
molecular mimicry, 47, 120
monocytes, 57, 82, 134
Morning Glory syndrome, 12, 37
mucosal-associated lymphoid tissue
  (MALT), 22, 81, 90
Müller cells, 53, 128
muscle fibres, extraocular, 91
mutations, 21, 89–90
mydriasis, 129
mydriatic agents, 54, 129
myopia, simple, 51, 126
myotonic dystrophy, 58, 135

Na^+/K^+ ATPase pump, 14, 52, 81,
  127
naevus, junctional, 79
nasociliary nerve, 3, 74
nasolacrimal groove, 108–9
nasopharyngeal carcinoma, 115
natural killer (NK) cells, 82
neck, anterior triangle, 36, 108
necrotizing vasculitis, 40, 113
Neisseria, 92
neural crest, 36, 108
  cranial, 22, 91
neural crest cells, 41, 114
  migration, 108
neuroectoderm, 5, 91

neurofibromatosis, 82
neurohypophysis, 57, 134
neurones, neurosecretory, 28, 99
neutropenia, 47, 121
neutrophils, 15, 82
  granulocytes, 28, 98
NMDA receptors, 87
non-parametric statistical tests, 132
non-steroidal anti-inflammatory
    drugs (NSAIDs), 25, 94
nonsense mutation, 21, 89
noradrenaline, 134
nucleic acid synthesis inhibitors,
    63, 141
nucleotides, cyclic, 99
null hypothesis, 54, 129–30
nystagmus, vertical, 30, 101–2

occipital cortex V4 region, 52,
    127
occipital sinuses, 5, 69–70
occipital visual area, 131
ocular neovascularization, 11, 78
oculomotor nerve, 3, 67
onchocerciasis, 47, 120
ophthalmic artery, 44, 82, 118
opponent theory, 52, 127
optic canal, 118
optic chiasm, 4, 6, 41, 72
  compression, 113
optic disk, 12, 79
  rods, 129
optic nerve, 6, 71
  6-week-old embryo, 72
  development, 37, 110
  glioma, 15, 82
  hypoplasia, 52, 127
  meningioma, 82
  myelination, 6, 46, 72, 120
  trisomy 13, 127
optic tracts, 35, 107
orbit, 3, 46, 120
  lateral wall, 42, 114
orbital margin, 7, 73
oscillopsia, 101–2
otic ganglion, 60, 137

p24 antigenaemia, 79
P_{450} drug-metabolizing system, 55,
    130
parametric tests, 25, 94
parasympathetic activity blockade,
    28, 98
parasympathetic fibres, 3, 107
parathyroid gland, 37, 109
  inferior, 110
parvocellular system, 20, 52, 89,
    127
Patau syndrome, 52, 127
penicillin, 43
  allergy, 141
  resistance, 3
peptidyl transferase inhibition, 141
petrosal nerve, deep, 96
petrosal sinuses, 4, 5, 69–70
phagocytes, 82, 95
pharyngeal arch, 110
  development, 10, 77
  first, 6, 10, 38, 72, 77, 110, 120
  fourth, 38, 109, 110, 120
  second, 10, 37, 46, 109, 120
  sixth, 10
  third, 38, 109, 110, 120
phenylephrine, 57, 129, 134
phosphatidyl inositol, 61, 138
phospholipase A_2, 55, 61, 131, 139
photoreceptors
  atrophy, 41, 114
  inner segment, 102, 128
  outer segment, 29, 100
physostigmine, 129
pigmentation, tissue, 38, 111
  melanin, 40, 112
pilocarpine, 94
pituicytes, 134
pituitary gland, 134
platelet-derived growth factor, 62,
    140
platelets, 9
plexiform layer, outer, 74
point mutation, 89
polymerase chain reaction (PCR),
    31, 51, 102, 125

polymorphonuclear leucocytes, 38,
110
polymorphonuclear leucocytic
infiltrate, 15, 83
polymorphs, 57, 82, 134
polysaccharide degradation, 130
posterior communicating artery, 3,
67
postsynaptic motor endplate, 27, 97
potassium, corneal, 52, 127
procaine, 100
proliferation, reactionary, 38, 111
prostaglandins, 99
psammoma bodies, 15, 82
pterygopalatine ganglion, 88
ptosis, 3
pulmonary arterioles, embolic
disease, 9, 75
pupillary membrane formation, 41,
114
pupils, 21
dilatation, 134, 135
Holmes–Adie syndrome, 90
purines, 89
pyrimidines, 89

quinolones, 141

rami lacrimales, 88
red cells
inclusions, 63, 140–1
lysis, 136
renin secretion stimulation, 56, 132
restriction endonuclease enzymes,
51, 125
reticular fibres, lymph nodes, 95
reticulocytes, 63, 140
retina
arterial supply, 11, 77–8
development, 42, 114, 120
differentiation, 6, 46, 120
Müller cells, 53, 128
nerve fibre layer atrophy, 41,
114
neurosensory, 128–9
retinal detachment, 41, 113

retinal disk, 91
retinal dysplasia, 52, 127
retinal ganglion cells, 20, 88–9
retinal pigment epithelium, 28, 55,
99, 128
Bruch's membrane, 53, 128
cells, 54, 130
retinitis pigmentosa, 41, 113
retinoblastoma, 82
hereditary, 51, 89, 126
retro-orbital plexus, 88
rhodopsin, 58, 100, 135
ribosomes, 91
rickettsial infection, 63, 141
right fourth nerve nucleus, 4, 69
right superior oblique, 4
river blindness, 47, 120
RNA viruses, 12, 42, 79, 118
rods, 53, 128–9
rough endoplasmic reticulum, 91–2
roundworm infestations, 4, 68

sarcoidosis, 39, 111
Schiotz tonometer, 60, 137
sclera, 5, 44, 70, 117
mesoderm derivative, 46, 120
serine protease inhibitors, 58, 136
short stature, 51, 125
sialyl transferase, 93
siderocytes, 63, 140
skull development, 43, 116
sodium, 52
corneal, 127
renal reabsorption, 132
sodium channels, 100
inhibition, 139
somatomedin, 28, 99
somatostatin, 28, 99
Southern blotting, 51, 125
sphenoid bone, 42, 81, 110
spider venom, 97
spina recti lateralis, 42, 114
stapes, 46, 109, 120
Staphylococcus aureus, 3, 44, 45, 68,
117, 118
Stargardt's dystrophy, 51, 126

statistical tests
  confidence intervals, 62, 140
  non-parametric, 56, 132
  null hypothesis, 54, 129–30
  parametric tests, 25, 94
stem cells, 59, 136
sterilization, autoclave, 31, 103
steroid sex hormones, 99
Stickler's syndrome, 51, 125
stop codon, 89
straight sinuses, 5, 69–70
streptococci, β haemolytic, 36, 42, 115
Streptococcus pneumoniae, 36, 108
striate cortex, 6
Student's t test, 25, 94, 132
stylohyoid ligament, 109
stylopharyngeus, 6, 72, 120
sulphonamides, 62, 103, 139
superficial temporal artery, 112
superior oblique muscle, 37, 110
superior orbital fissure, 3, 67
suxamethonium, 62, 140
sweat gland innervation, 98
syphilis, 39, 111
systemic disease, 39, 111
systemic lupus erythematosus (SLE), 39, 40, 111, 113

T cells, 9, 25, 26, 58, 75, 95, 135
  antigen presentation, 55, 131
  cross-reactive antigen recognition, 120
  subsets, 31, 103–4
t-test, 25, 94, 132
Takayasu's disease, 40, 113
tarsal plate, 81
Tay–Sachs disease, 41, 114
tear film, 15, 82–3
  characteristics, 26, 96
  structure, 20, 88
temporal arteritis, 40, 113
Tenon's capsule, 46, 120
tensor palati, 60, 137
tensor tympani, 60, 137
termination codon, 89

tetracaine, 100
tetracyclines, 27, 96–7
thalamus, 71
thiazide diuretics, 24, 93–4
thioglycolate broth, 92
thyroid cartilage, 6, 120
tonometer, non-contact, 137
tonsils, epithelial lining, 37, 109
toxic shock syndrome, 44, 117
Toxocara canis, 4, 68
toxoplasmosis, 43, 116
transforming growth factor β, 99
transitions, 21, 89
translation, genetic code, 126
transverse sinuses, 5, 69–70
transversion, 21, 89
Treacher Collins syndrome, 43, 116
Trichinella spiralis, 4, 68
trichromatic theory, 52, 127
tricyclic antidepressants, 58, 135
trigeminal nerve
  first division, 8, 74
  pharyngeal arch, 77
trisomy 13, 52, 127
tritanopia, 51, 125
trochlear nerve, 4
trophozoites, 80
tropomyosin, 130
troponin, 130
tumour necrosis factor α (TNF-α), 58, 135
tumours
  benign, 12, 79
  epithelial cell, 39, 112
  malignant soft-tissue, 40, 112–13
  see also metastases
Turner syndrome, 51, 125

universal code, 126
uridine triphosphate, 56, 132

vagal tone blockade, 98
vancomycin, 53, 127–8
varicella zoster virus, 57, 133
vascular endothelial growth factor (VEGF), 11, 78

venous sinuses, paired, 5, 69–70
vertebral arteries, 45, 119
vimentin, 54, 130
virulence factors, 108
visual evoked potential, 55, 130–1
vitamin A, 27, 58, 97, 135
vitamin K, 60
vitreous, 7, 73
  cavity, 30, 101
  development, 37, 109
  gel, 28, 98–9
  persistent hyperplastic primary, 52, 127
vitronectin, 58, 136

warfarin, 60, 138
wavelength discrimination, 127
Wegener's granulomatosis, 40, 113

X-linked diseases, 19, 22, 59, 87, 91, 136
  dominant inheritance, 22, 91
  recessive, 59, 136

Young–Helmholtz trichromatic theory, 52, 127

zygomatic foramen, 114
zygomatic nerve, 114
zygomatic vessels, 114